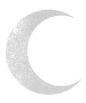

# THE NATURAL
# SLEEPER

### A Bedside Guide to Complementary
### and Alternative Solutions for Better Sleep

## JULIE WRIGHT

## TILLER PRESS
New York   London   Toronto   Sydney   New Delhi

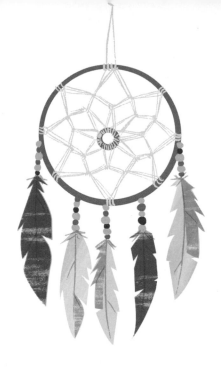

TILLER PRESS

An Imprint of Simon & Schuster, Inc.
1230 Avenue of the Americas
New York, NY 10020

First Tiller Press trade paperback edition March 2021

TILLER PRESS and colophon are trademarks of Simon &
Schuster, Inc.

For information about special discounts for bulk
purchases, please contact Simon & Schuster Special Sales
at 1-866-506-1949 or business@simonandschuster.com.

The Simon & Schuster Speakers Bureau can bring
authors to your live event. For more information or
to book an event, contact the Simon & Schuster
Speakers Bureau at 1-866-248-3049 or visit our website
at www.simonspeakers.com.

Interior design by Rachel Cross

Manufactured in China

10  9  8  7  6  5  4  3  2  1

Library of Congress Cataloging-in-Publication Data
has been applied for.

ISBN 978-1-9821-6065-4
ISBN 978-1-9821-6069-2 (ebook)

# A NOTE ON SAFETY

When followed carefully and regularly, the advice and instructions in *The Natural Sleeper* can have a beneficial effect on sleep. Ideally progress slowly, implementing one change at a time and observe any results before safely proceeding to the next one. If you notice undesirable side effects, discomfort, pain, difficulties, or any adverse reactions, please stop immediately and consult with your professional health provider or doctor.

You are encouraged to first discuss any new treatment, therapy, or practice with your healthcare provider (medical doctor or primary care physician) before following the suggested advice, especially anything you ingest, such as foods, herbal remedies, supplements, or nutrients; anything you inhale, such as essential oils; any form of physical practice, such as exercise and movement; any form of psychological practice or therapy; or any electric or electronic devices, such as gadgets and artificial light. This is because, while unlikely, there is a possibility these may have a negative effect on your physical or mental health and have harmful or neutralizing interactions with other medicine you are taking.

Seek medical advice, especially if you have any existing health conditions and allergies, if you are pregnant or breastfeeding, if you are under the age of 18, or if you are already taking any medication, supplements, or herbal remedies. You should also seek medical help if your sleep issue has been going on for longer than a few months.

Following the advice and instructions from this book is the reader's decision and responsibility. Its author and publisher are not liable for any errors or omissions. By reading and following instructions and advice in this book, the reader indemnifies the author from any results or consequences, even if negative or harmful. *The Natural Sleeper* is not a substitute for medical advice.

# CONTENTS

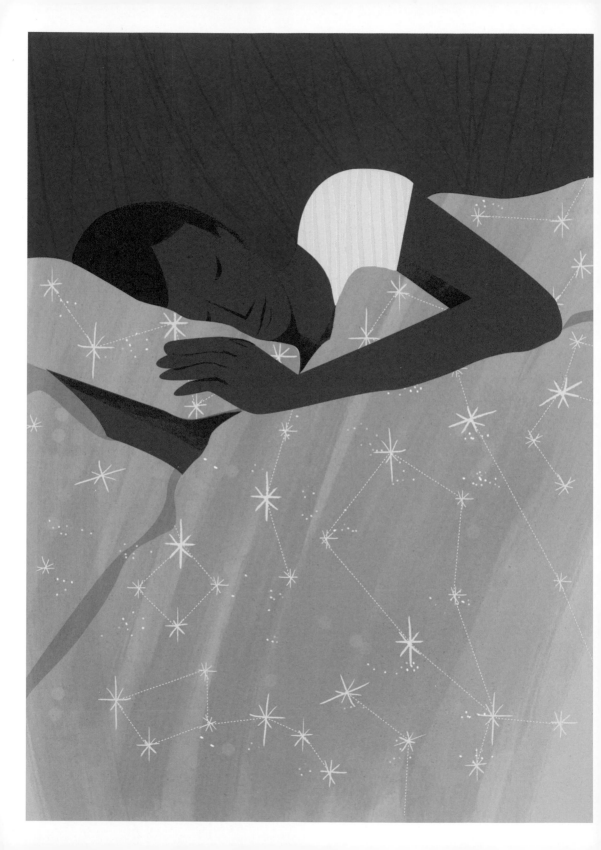

# INTRODUCTION

Welcome to *The Natural Sleeper: A Bedside Guide to Complementary and Alternative Solutions for Better Sleep*. This book starts with an easy-to-understand introduction to sleep, followed by a wide range of natural solutions, therapies, techniques, habits, and tips to help improve your sleep. Before I introduce myself, allow me to first give you some context and perspective on this essential human need.

## THE CONTEXT

Public awareness about the impact of sleep deprivation and insomnia is at an all-time high. Sleep medicine and psychological support for sleep are finally at the forefront of the physical and mental health debate. Is it because an increasing number of us experience difficulties falling or staying asleep? Is it because more medical studies are emerging showing a correlation between sleep deprivation and serious medical conditions? Is it because the media is now much more focused on sleep as an aspect of wellness?

In recent years, it seems as if sleep is finally being recognized as a supporting pillar for health, rather than being viewed as a time-consuming inconvenience. Sleep has been identified as a key factor in the prevention and cure of many mental and physical illnesses, and as a foundation for our happiness, balance, and natural functioning. Glorifying the need for only a short amount of sleep is no longer fashionable, nor a proof of being a superhuman.

According to a study by the Centers for Disease Control and Prevention (CDC), more than one-third of American adults are not getting enough sleep on a regular basis[1]. Meanwhile, a poll conducted by the National Sleep Foundation (NSF) found that "more than half of the people interviewed reported at least one symptom of insomnia a few nights per week within the past year" and "thirty-three percent said they had at least one of these symptoms every night or almost every night in the past year."[2] According to a RAND Corporation study, every year sleep deprivation is costing the US economy about 1.23 million working days, translating into a loss of $411 billion, or 2.28 percent of GDP.[3]

Sleeping is meant to be as easy as breathing. We should not have to work hard at it because it is a natural built-in process. Our physiology as humans has not fundamentally been altered, so what has changed? Scientists and psychologists report a range of factors:

+ An increasing amount of artificial lighting confusing our brains as to when it is time to be asleep or awake.
+ Increasing stimulation levels in an always-on connected environment and

an accelerating pace of change, with growing pressure and expectations.

+ Fewer environmental threats (think saber-toothed tigers), but perhaps more complex problems to solve and more ongoing threatening psychological events generating stress and fear.

+ Being on a journey of constant learning and adaptation due to the fast-paced technological advancements we have to keep up with. It is likely that we are processing more data and information today requiring more brain power and management.

+ Our irregular and demanding lifestyles making it hard to honor routines over performance.

## MEET JULIE WRIGHT

As a sleep educator and ambassador, I founded WeSleep with the mission to help people live better lives by improving their sleep naturally. My motto is: "Sleep, and your dreams will come true." I work with sleep scientists and therapists to deliver learning sessions, experiential workshops, talks, webinars, and one-to-one consultations. Whether in a private setting or at the workplace, we preach sleep through education and practical exercises, taster sessions and demonstrations, actionable tips, and product recommendations.

I see myself as an enabler and a passionate messenger, connecting people who struggle with sleep with people who can help them. While academics and scientists share their knowledge often as observers, my point of view combines practical experience and experimentation as a former insomniac, who still goes through sleepless phases from time to time.

Sleep seems to be a much more complex process compared to losing weight or building strength and endurance. As a sleep practitioner, I want to take you on a journey of discovery, education, inspiration, and healing because I know too well about the negative impact of sleep deprivation, having battled with sleep issues myself. I have researched the subject for 8 years, surrounding myself with long-standing academic experts—something I still do every day. I embarked on a journey filled with learning, extensive research, and therapeutic experimentation, which I would like to share in this book. Armed with theoretical knowledge, it was important to me to try, test, and experiment with a wide array of natural solutions, therapies, medicinal systems, and techniques to find better sleep.

Experimenting is truly the answer because everyone is different, and every night can be different, too. It is about being inspired by a wide range of perspectives, contemporary or ancient, from various cultures, and different approaches, whether scientific, spiritual, empirical, behavioral, or remedy-based.

Sleep is like an orchestra, with musicians and instruments. And the brain is its maestro. To adapt, adjust, and respond, you need to gather your own bag of tricks, tools, and solutions.

The Natural Sleeper is the result of my findings and an opportunity for you to pause, reflect, try new things, and walk away with your personal sleep strategy so that you can become reenergized by learning how to sleep naturally for optimal physical and mental health. Most importantly, don't ignore insomnia or sleep deprivation. Whether it's long term, or whether you happen to be going through a rough patch, the impact of not getting enough sleep is underestimated. With a good night's sleep, nothing can stop you, and you will most likely be able to achieve your dreams. I believe good sleep can help you be superhuman.

If you'd like to join the conversation about sleep, have further questions, or are interested in additional resources to actively improve your sleep, visit www.thenaturalsleeper.com or email me at julie@thenaturalsleeper.com. I will personally respond to all emails and help you make the most of this book by helping you navigate it according to your own personal circumstances.

## ABOUT THIS BOOK

The Natural Sleeper is an introduction to an extensive range of natural methods, therapies, and alternative solutions to achieve better sleep and manage bouts of insomnia. "Natural" can be defined in many ways, but in this book I am talking about non-medicated options, staying away from sleeping pills, prescriptions, and pharmaceuticals.

There is a wealth of information and tips in The Natural Sleeper, but fear not, each article was written simply and gives you a straightforward overview and basic explanation about each topic.

The two charts on the following pages are navigation guides to help you find the remedies and therapies most suited to your specific needs. Look at the charts and see where each therapy or solution is positioned on the axes: the further away a dot is positioned from the center, the higher it is in terms of scale and/or intensity for this particular criteria.

Think about yourself and the criteria you relate to the most. Then locate the corresponding suggestions in each quadrant. You can then refer to their page or section for an explanation and further details. For example, if you are someone who's reasonably patient and are not sleeping because your mind is restless at night, you could explore mind management techniques. Or if you are someone who is looking for solutions that you can execute on your own, and if you are more on the practical side, you may want to explore wind down practices and building your cocoon.

We are complex beings, so you may relate to many criteria all at once, or some may make more sense during certain periods of your life. So be flexible, use common sense, and experiment.

# FIND A SLEEP SOLUTION FOR YOU   SELF-CARE

"**Intuitive**" means therapies or solutions that lean toward one or more of the following characteristics: abstract, energy-based, mind-body connection, sensory, experimental, belief-based, spiritual practice, or healing. It's about what you sense and feel, and sometimes beyond the visible and scientifically proven.

"**Pragmatic**" means therapies or solutions that feel more practical, rational, concrete, material, or behavioral. It's about what you do on a more practical level.

MARMA POINTS THERAPY (P.122)   MINDFULNESS (P.78)

MUDRAS (P.80)

TAI CHI AND QIGONG (P.100)   VISUALIZATION (P.81)

MEDITATION (P.78)

## INTUITIVE

SPIRITUAL PRACTICES (P.94)

AROMATHERAPY (P.170)

YOGA NIDRA (P.75)

FLOWER ESSENCES (P.168)

AUTOGENICS (P.93)

SOPHROLOGY (P.94)

HOMEOPATHY (P.126)

AYURVEDA (P.120)   ACUPUNCTURE (P.131)

ENERGY-HEALING THERAPIES (P.141)   BODY-BASED THERAPIES (P.135)

TRADITIONAL CHINESE MEDICINE (P.128)   PSYCHO-EMOTIONAL HEALING THERAPIES (P.92)

HYPNOTHERAPY (P.92)

## PROFESSIONAL SUPPORT

SELF-CARE

"Self-care" means what you can do pretty much on your own.

"Professional support" means that you are likely to need the guidance of a professional therapist, doctor, or instructor—at least initially.

WIND-DOWN PRACTICES
AND RITUALS (P.40)

BUILDING
YOUR
COCOON
(P.52)

HYDRATION AND
DRINKS (P.115)

SLEEP POSITIONS
(P.83)

MANAGING
JET LAG (P.71)

LIGHTS ROUTINE (P.67)

SLEEP TECHNOLOGY
(P.177)

APPS (P.183)

MIND-FOCUS
TECHNIQUES (P.82)

EXERCISE AND GENTLE
MOVEMENT (P.97)

SOUND THERAPY
(P.149)

MIND-MANAGEMENT
TECHNIQUES (P.87)

PROGRESSIVE MUSCLE RELAXATION
AND BODY SCAN (P.78)

BREATHWORK
(P.76)

PRAGMATIC

CBD (P.167)

LIGHT THERAPY (P.69)

NEUROACOUSTICS (P.150)

MUSIC THERAPY
(P.156)

HERBAL REMEDIES (P.161)

NUTRITIONAL
HEALING (P.103)

CONTACT-BASED
THERAPIES (P.144)

CBTI (P.188)

SOUND BATHS
(P.156)

WATER-BASED THERAPIES (P.138)

TALK THERAPIES (P.95)

PROFESSIONAL SUPPORT

MIND | PSYCHOLOGICAL

"Mind/Psychological" relates to mental therapies or solutions that require the brain and the mind to be fully involved in the healing and well-being process. These can have a psychological and/or physiological effect.

"Environment/Physical" relates to the therapies or solutions that have a more pragmatic impact on the body, lean towards more material approaches, or are designed to improve the environment in which we live to facilitate sleep.

"Immediate impact" means that the results should be felt quickly, either immediately, or within days to a couple of weeks.

"Medium- to long-term results" means that it may take longer to observe significant changes in sleeping patterns, but these tend to be durable if they work for you.

MEDITATION (P.78)

HYPNOTHERAPY (P.92)

MINDFULNESS (P.78)

MIND FOCUS TECHNIQUES (P.82)

MARMA POINTS THERAPY (P.122)

VISUALIZATION (P.81)

TRADITIONAL CHINESE MEDICINE (P.128)

WIND DOWN PRACTICES AND RITUALS (P.40)

NEUROACOUSTICS (P.150)

IMMEDIATE IMPACT

SOUND THERAPY (P.149)

BREATHWORK (P.76)

PROGRESSIVE MUSCLE RELAXATION AND BODY SCAN (P.78)

AUTOGENICS (P.93)

YOGA NIDRA (P.75)

SOUND BATHS (P.156)

BODY-BASED THERAPIES (P.135)

EXERCISE AND GENTLE MOVEMENT (P.97)

SLEEP POSITIONS (P.83)

CONTACT-BASED THERAPIES (P.144)

MANAGING JET LAG (P.71)

HYDRATION AND DRINKS (P.115)

SLEEP TECHNOLOGY (P.177)

BUILDING YOUR COCOON (P.52)

LIGHTS ROUTINE (P.67)

ENVIRONMENT | PHYSICAL

MIND I PSYCHOLOGICAL

TALK THERAPIES (P.95)

MIND-MANAGEMENT
TECHNIQUES (P.87)

PSYCHO-EMOTIONAL
HEALING THERAPIES (P.92)          CBTI (P.188)

• SOPHROLOGY (P.94)

SPIRITUAL PRACTICES
(P.94)

MUDRAS          ENERGY-HEALING
(P.80)          THERAPIES (P.141)

FLOWER ESSENCES
(P.168)

AYURVEDA (P.120)

HOMEOPATHY (P.126)

MEDIUM- TO LONG-
TERM RESULTS

WATER-BASED THERAPIES
(P.138)

AROMATHERAPY (P.170)

CBD (P.167)

HERBAL REMEDIES (P.161)

TAI CHI AND QIGONG (P.100)

APPS (P.183)

NUTRITIONAL HEALING (P.103)

MUSIC THERAPY (P.156)

LIGHT THERAPY (P.69)

ENVIRONMENT I PHYSICAL

# UNDERSTANDING SLEEP

## WHY SHOULD WE CARE? THE IMPACT OF SLEEP DEPRIVATION

We intuitively know and feel from our personal experience that sleep is good for us, further validating the scientific advice. Some of the negative consequences of sleep deprivation are obvious, while others are initially hidden and insidious. Sleep loss can be the direct cause of some medical or psychological conditions, or it may be correlated but not necessarily the cause. Either way, there is a bidirectional link between sleep and health, which we should not underestimate.

What we do know is that a lack of sleep leads to poorer mental and physical performance, and a lower ability to concentrate, focus, reason, make good assessments or decisions, and solve problems. Unfortunately, this results in an impaired capacity to learn new things or access memories. Sleep deprivation weakens our immune system, impacts our fertility, makes us irritable, and causes us to feel down, giving us a negative outlook on the day. It affects our appetite (generally increasing it), our motivation and willpower, and our exercise regime. We are likely to become more accident prone, more lethargic, and less proactive. By not getting enough sleep we are 3 to 5 times more likely to become depressed. Our ability to cope with stress and deal with pressurized situations is diminished. There are also serious long-term medical consequences of sleep deprivation, which have been scientifically linked to diseases such as cardiovascular illnesses, obesity, diabetes, Alzheimer's disease, and some forms of cancer.

## THE IMPORTANCE OF SLEEP

On the flipside, prioritizing sleep can lead to such positive outcomes and improve your life, setting you up for happiness and success. Quality sleep can help in so many ways, including:

+ Increased energy and motivation.
+ Improved mind clarity, learning, problem-solving, and productivity.
+ More enthusiasm for social interaction.
+ Improved mood.
+ Feeling and looking more attractive.
+ Being healthier physically and mentally.

The list goes on, so what's not to like? By prioritizing sleep and recovery, you are supporting your body, brain, and mind, and respecting and optimizing your natural rhythms and processes for a stronger and better version of yourself. Your brain and body need rest, recovery, and sleep to fire neurons properly, synchronize organs, coordinate physiological processes, and repair muscles and tissues. The overwhelming evidence is that sleeping well can be a huge support to your health and well-being—in fact, sleep is their foundation.

## WHY SLEEP SHOULD MATTER TO YOU

If understanding the importance of sleep and the impact of sleep deprivation is still not enough of an incentive, reflect on what a lack of sleep is costing you, personally. It could be your health, your relationship, your career, your weight and figure, your finances, your attractiveness, your fertility. Ask yourself, "What could be better in my life if only I slept more and better?" Think about the positive changes you could create, the achievements you could aim for. It is important to find your specific personal motivation, leading you on a journey of discovery and commitment toward peaceful slumber.

# FUNDAMENTALS AND BASICS ABOUT SLEEP

Sleep could be explained in a few sentences, yet that would not do it justice because it is a complex and fascinating subject. Some aspects of sleep remain a mystery, even for the most knowledgeable scientists and researchers. In fact, even if experts have a good idea of what happens during sleep, no one seems to be sure why we must sleep, biologically speaking. Fortunately, the volume of clinical and research studies about sleep and insomnia is increasing and the public is now paying attention. Rather than a deep dive into the science of sleep, this section provides some basic knowledge and fundamentals that will help your understanding throughout the rest of the book. Note that some topics addressed in this chapter are covered in more detail later in the book.

## WHY DO WE SLEEP?

Sleep is a biological enigma, but based on what scientists have observed, it appears that it is needed to repair and maintain our physical and mental functions and that sleep quality and quantity are as important to our health as breathing, drinking, eating, and moving.

What is certain is that we are designed to sleep for roughly one-third of our lives, which means that, with a life expectancy of 78.54 years in the US, we will have slept just over 215,000 hours on average during our time on planet Earth.

Even if sleep cannot be fully explained, the negative consequences and risks linked to sleep loss or deprivation are clear and tangible. This should be enough to make sleep a priority in your life. As independent sleep expert Dr. Neil Stanley says, "Sleep is a biological need, not an inconvenience."

## SLUMBER MAGIC

During sleep, our brain, cells, organs, tissues, and bones recover, heal, grow, cleanse, and reset. Without sleep our memory, data and information processing, and learning abilities would be impaired.

True magic happens while we are asleep. Our brain goes through one of its most essential daily phases: It processes data, information, and emotions; cleanses itself from harmful toxins; and consolidates and stabilizes new learning and memory, deciding what to store, file, or delete. The human growth hormone, essential for growing and repairing our bodies from daily injury, is released while we are unconscious, making each hour of sleep count.

Our endocrine, metabolic, and immune systems depend on sleep for optimal functioning. Our mood, motivation, and energy levels are much improved with a good night's sleep. Our cardiovascular health is also optimized with sufficient quality sleep.

## SLEEP STAGES

Our sleep goes through several cycles, each made up of four stages that are slightly different in duration and purpose. Each sleep cycle lasts on average 90 minutes and is made up of non-rapid eye movement (NREM) sleep (stages N1–N3) and rapid eye movement (REM) sleep. We are either in NREM sleep (75 percent of the night) or REM sleep (25 percent of the night).

- N1 is the lightest stage, between our awake and sleep state, which we can easily be woken up from. Our muscles may twitch, contracting and releasing rapidly, perhaps giving a sense of falling or tripping. Our nervous system switches from active to fully relaxed (see page 22).
- N2 is light sleep when unconsciousness begins, during which the body temperature drops, and our blood pressure, breathing, and heart rate start to slow down.
- N3 is deep sleep, also called slow-wave sleep (SWS) or delta sleep, a time during which the body repairs and grows. This is the restorative sleep that makes you feel alert, refreshed, and rested in the morning. Our brain waves are at their slowest and human growth hormone is released. It is believed that SWS plays a major role in learning and memory consolidation, too.
- REM is the rapid eye movement phase during which our brain is active again, as if we are awake. Our eyes motion quickly back and forth. This is when we dream, but our muscles are switched off and paralyzed, so we do not act out our dreams. During this state we process emotions, manifest creativity, solve problems, and further consolidate our learning and memory, retaining what is useful and relevant.

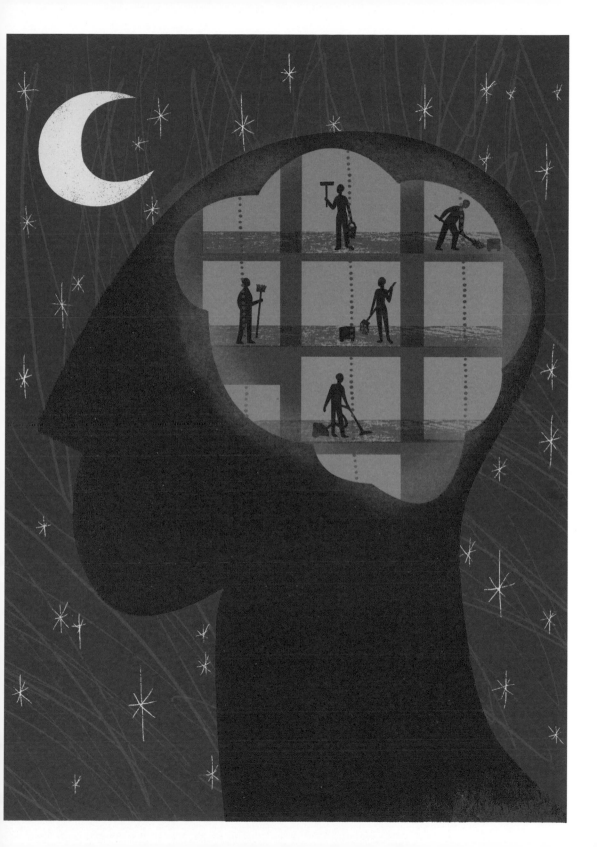

Each REM sleep stage lengthens throughout the night, so that most of REM sleep occurs during the second part of the night.

NREM and REM sleep alternate 5 to 6 times every night, resulting in 5 to 6 cycles on average. The first 3 cycles in the first 4 to 5 hours are necessary simply to function the next day. The last 1 to 2 cycles are essential to optimize our physical and mental functioning. REM stages gradually get longer throughout the night, while our SWS (deep) stages get shorter. It is okay and quite normal to wake up periodically during the night for a few seconds or a few minutes, as long as you can fall back to sleep easily. This is likely explained by ancestral requirements to wake up regularly to check our surroundings for predators.

The general recommendation is to have, on average, 7 to 8 hours sleep per night, starting with deeper and more restorative deep sleep and ending with more of the lighter REM sleep, essential for our psychological well-being. That said, the length of sleep we need depends on our individual genetic requirements and can be as low as 4 to 5 hours and as high as 10 to 11 hours, although both are extreme cases. The recommendations for sleep duration can be found on page 32.

## THE NATURAL SLEEP–WAKE PROCESS

To sleep well, you must first understand how our brains and bodies work, influencing each other to make us fall asleep or wake up. The execution of a sleep–wake cycle is complex and is the result of carefully orchestrated and sequenced processes: Exposure to natural light rules a master clock ensuring regular timings; the production and release of specific hormones and neurotransmitters working for us at the right time of the day and night; our natural pressure to sleep builds up during the day and depletes while we sleep; and finally our nervous system acts as an on-off switch, activating or relaxing us at the right time. If anything goes wrong in

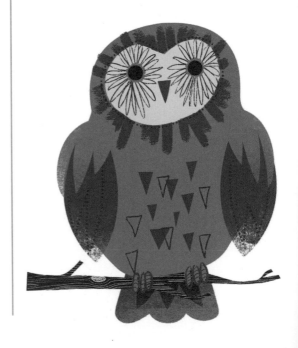

this coordinated chain of events, we are unlikely to sleep well.

We must optimize our environment, physical health, physiological condition, and psychological state of mind to create the perfect conditions for a good night's sleep. We should do so in a regular and rhythmic fashion, ensuring balance, preparation, and safety and, most importantly, make the time to sleep.

## ENVIRONMENTAL FACTORS

The key environmental factors that influence our sleep are light, temperature, comfort, and noise levels. We are diurnal beings by nature, which means that we should be active during the day and rest at night. Natural sunlight is as essential to us as darkness. Environmental factors help our brain understand whether it is time to be active or rest. Darkness reduces the level of visual stimulation we experience. Loud daytime noises fading away (to be replaced by more gentle nocturnal noises) lessen brain stimulation. Similarly, a temperature drop indicates the night coming, which has a direct physiological impact on us in preparation for sleep. A number of hormonal processes respond to the presence or absence of sunlight, routinely alternating, regularly and rhythmically. Finally, settling into a comfortable and cozy nest or cocoon (see pages 53-63) completes the perfect set up for slumber.

## INTERNAL PROCESSES

So how does this translate into specific physiological processes in our brain and body?

Our body's internal clock, or circadian rhythm, is our natural time machine for sleep. Its scientific name is the suprachiasmatic nucleus (SCN), which is a tiny region of the brain in the hypothalamus, located right behind our eyes. It is responsive to sunlight and responsible for instructing the release of natural sleep-inducing chemicals in our bodies. It runs in approximately 24-hour cycles alongside light–darkness cycles and differentiates daytime from nighttime, which helps us manages our life cycles. This is why it is so important to maintain a regular day–night routine: When to sleep, when to eat, when to be active, when to relax. Imagine if you had a watch and kept playing with the small and big hands, then tried to figure out what time it truly is?

The homeostatic sleep drive, or sleep pressure, is an internal biochemical system that not only counts time, but builds up the feeling of being sleepy, until you are no longer able to stay awake. The pressure to sleep then decreases as you sleep so you can wake up in due time. This process works hand in hand with the circadian rhythm, whereby the body clock is the timekeeper (= when) and the sleep homeostatic process is the sleepiness indicator (= how much). If you feel like you are going to have a "good night's sleep," it indicates that your sleep pressure has built up sufficiently. Also be aware that napping will deplete your sleep pressure, especially if you are chronically sleep deprived, which means that you are less likely to sleep sufficiently that night.

The central nervous system plays a critical role in getting us to switch off and sleep. It is split in two: The sympathetic nervous system is the "doing" part that helps you get up and go or run away from stressful or dangerous situations. It is triggered automatically in "fight or flight" situations, typically happening during the daytime. It is also responsible for stimulating the release of the stress hormones adrenaline and cortisol. Nervous fatigue occurs when we are exhausted, but the sympathetic nervous system is fully switched on due to stress, for example.

The second part is the parasympathetic nervous system, which enables you to relax and get to sleep in the first place. To be able to sleep, your sympathetic nervous system needs to slow down. One way to do this is to activate the vagus nerve, which is a sort of on-off switch. It runs from your stomach to the throat and the back of the brain. When activated, the body flips from the sympathetic over to the parasympathetic nervous system. It is more easily activated when your breathing is deep and relaxed, for example with abdominal breathing (see pages 76-77).

## SLEEP HORMONES, OUR NATURAL SLEEPING PILLS

The endocrine system is complex, and there are three essential agents helping us fall asleep and wake up. The human body has an internal pharmacy of natural neurochemicals helping regulate our sleep-wake cycles.

Cortisol, the "fight or flight" hormone, is released under stress and helps us run away from danger, but it is also a great "get up and go" hormone released early morning to prompt us to wake up; it also helps us perform during intense exercise and sports activities. Without cortisol we would struggle to make a start each day. It is important to "spend" your cortisol hormones by being active throughout the day—if a surplus remains in your body overnight when you are meant to be sleeping, it will undoubtedly create sleep disruptions.

Serotonin, the happy hormone, is produced from a combination of certain foods containing tryptophan (see page 111) and exposure to sunlight, which helps us absorb the vitamin D that is essential to produce serotonin. Some 90 to 95 percent of serotonin is created in the gut from the food we eat. It then goes through metabolic changes to transform into melatonin when it reaches the pineal gland in the brain. Serotonin is therefore a precursor to melatonin.

Melatonin helps regulate the body's circadian rhythm and promotes restful sleep. It is produced and released starting

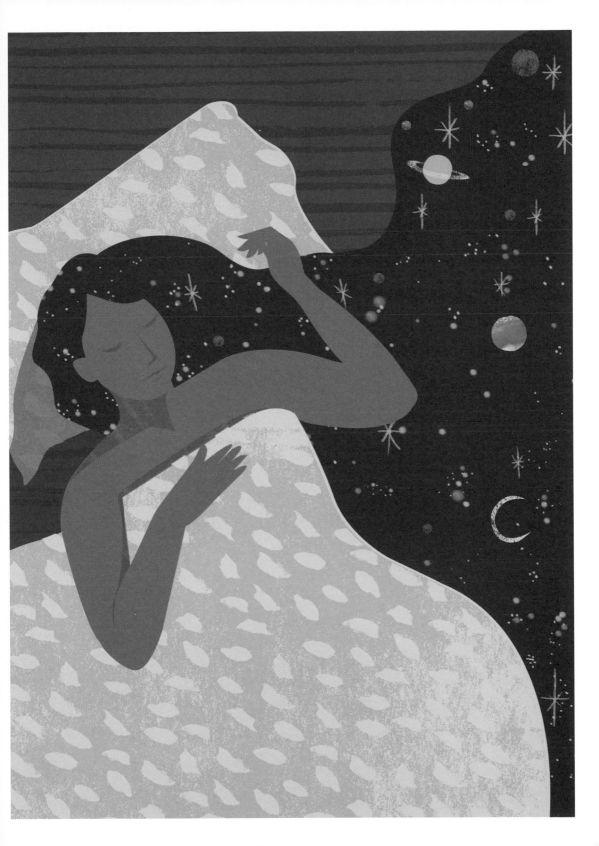

in the afternoon into the night, prompted by a signal from the eyes to the brain, when the sunlight level starts to decrease. It then peaks in the early hours of the morning. At sunrise, our SCN (see page 21) perceives the start of daylight through our closed eyelids then suppresses the release of melatonin, making space for cortisol to take effect. See page 29 for information about melatonin supplements.

# DREAMS AND NIGHTMARES

While we are asleep, lying unconscious, we all dream on average 4 to 6 times every night, whether we remember our dreams or not. Dreams are a visual expression of the product of our brain accompanied by emotions, actions, perceived movements, thoughts, and sometimes sensations that are not real but feel real. Dreaming remains a scientific mystery, yet the best-known hypothesis is that it is therapeutic by helping us regulate emotions, especially negative ones such as fear, anxiety, anger, apprehension, and sadness, and sort the useful from the useless emotions. Our brain creates a memory of the experience linked to an emotion to reduce its power. Dreams prepare us for difficult situations, consolidate learnings, skills, and memories, and also activate our creativity and problem-solving abilities. Other theories are that through dreams we can:

- Relive and simulate a difficult situation in a safe context, thereby reducing its emotional impact and calming anxiety.
- Express ourselves and release repressed emotions.
- Train for and anticipate difficult real-life situations to come, experiencing them as if they were real, which helps us prepare should they happen.

*Note: Individuals who suffer from post-traumatic stress disorder (PTSD) struggle to benefit from the therapeutic effect of dreams, and instead suffer from nightmares, sadly unable to regulate painful emotions or forget them.*

## NEUROSCIENCE OF DREAMS, SIMPLIFIED

Dreams mostly occur during REM sleep when our body is paralyzed and we lose muscle tone so that we don't act out our dreams. Our amygdala, the emotion and fear region of the brain, is much more active and our rational front cortex in charge of reasoning is barely activated, which might explain the irrational nature of dreams. The regions of our brain light up in correlation with the events in our dreams, as if we were awake in real life. What we see and experience in our dreams is not real, but the emotions and sensations are, therefore our brain responds accordingly.

## PROFILE OF A DREAMER

On average, people remember 1 to 4 dreams each week, yet some claim they never dream. Why is this? Do heavy dreamers recall them more often, or is it that they dream more frequently? It is hard to say, but we know that they experience overnight awakenings twice as long as light dreamers (2 minutes versus 1 on average).[4] They seem more sensitive to their environment, experience more frequent sleep disruptions, and the brain region linked to alertness and external stimuli is more easily activated.

So, who is more likely to dream, or at least remember their dreams? The answer is people who are creative, explorers, seekers of new experiences, or those who suffer from anxiety.

There is a small category of individuals who are lucid dreamers, which means that they are aware and conscious that they are dreaming, and able to control the events and storyline. These dreamers claim they can solve problems, find inner peace, and reach higher consciousness. Lucid dreaming can be learned with patient practice, but is not generally recommended as it can disrupt natural sleep patterns.

## INTERPRETING OUR DREAMS

Our dreams can be positive or negative, but are mostly mundane and boring. We naturally tend to remember the bad, strange, or emotional ones more easily. There are many schools of interpretation going back to ancient times where dreams were thought to be messages from divine beings or signs foretelling the future. More recently Freudian theory claimed that dreams are expressions of self and a manifestation of repressed desires, wishes, and sexual needs. What most modern psychologists and neuroscientists believe is that dreams can only truly be interpreted by the dreamers themselves based on their life context and state of mind. A dream is often a mixture of real-life experiences, insignificant facts, and emotions. A repetitive or circumstantial dream, whether past or present, probably calls for your attention. How did you feel in your dream? Write it down as soon as you wake up (otherwise you risk forgetting within minutes) and think about your current life situation; specifically focus on the emotions felt in the dream rather than the events themselves.

## HOW TO DEAL WITH NIGHTMARES

A nightmare is different from a negative dream, although both occur during REM sleep. It is the product of intense fear, terror, distress, and anxiety accompanied by physical symptoms such as sweating, and an elevated heart rate and blood pressure. Nightmares are a normal reaction to stress for adults and should

## 7 BASIC PRINCIPLES FOR GOOD SLEEP

Having a good night's sleep will depend on the choices you make during the daytime and your ability to cope with the obstacles thrown in your way of good sleep. In theory, sleeping should be easy, as long as you follow these overarching principles:

1. Adopt daily sleep-promoting habits and lifestyle.

2. Ensure your body is healthy, well-nourished, and hydrated.

3. Keep your mind balanced and serene.

4. Maintain a rhythmic and regular routine.

5. Immerse yourself in a calm, safe, and sleep-inducing environment.

6. Respect your individual genetic predisposition in terms of when and how long to sleep.

7. Manage any medical condition, pain, or disorder causing sleep deprivation, whether directly or indirectly.

not be a major concern unless they happen frequently due to trauma or anxiety disorders. Having nightmares is normal for children up to 10 years old (it is part of their brain development) and more common for women than men. If you frequently experience distressing nightmares, here are some soothing methods worth trying:

+ First check with your doctor if the nightmares could be caused by prescription medicine, sleep apnea, ongoing sleep deprivation, depression, unhealthy habits, or abuse of drugs and stimulants.
+ Reflect consciously on the part of your life this nightmare calls attention for. Speak to a friend or therapist about it.
+ Confront your nightmare or difficult situation by gently recreating elements of its scenario in real life, adding one component at a time, only if it is safe, if you feel ready for it, and with good psychological support. It may help appease it.
+ Use a dream manipulation technique inspired by lucid dreamers, such as writing it down then rewriting the script while awake, changing one scene at a time to make it more comforting.
+ Explore other supervised techniques used for PTSD such as eye movement desensitization and reprocessing (EMDR) and Regenerating Images in Memory (RIM).
+ If you experience sleep paralysis, a temporary inability to move or speak

as you transition between sleep and awake states, you may feel very frightened, with the sensation of having a heavy weight on your chest leaving you breathless; your eyes might be able to move but not your body, and you may also have scary hallucinations. Firstly, know that sleep paralysis is not dangerous in any way and it will pass. It is best not to fight it; perhaps wiggle your toes and fingers for reassurance, clench your fists if you can, breathe very slowly without panicking. You may want to watch your sleep hygiene, especially adopting regular hours, avoiding any stimulants or foods before bedtime, and perhaps try CBTi (see page 88) as a helpful behavioral technique.

# WHY YOU MIGHT NOT BE SLEEPING WELL

To understand the possible reason(s) why you are not sleeping well, you must first understand the difference between the inability to sleep and the lack of opportunity to sleep. In the first instance you should seek professional help or try the self-help suggestions in this book. In the second instance, you should aim to take control of your daily activities and simply make sleep a life priority.

Loss of sleep or sleep deprivation is what defines insomnia. Whether short term or chronic, insomnia means having trouble falling asleep, waking up often during the night, or waking up too early and not being able to get back to sleep, all of which result in waking up feeling un-refreshed and with a less than optimal ability to function properly the next day.

The list of possible causes of insomnia is endless, since sleep is such a complex and precise process. In addition, some of the causes are unclear or need further scientific research to be validated. Possible contributing factors are highlighted throughout this book, along with suggested natural approaches, solutions, and therapies.

Some common causes for sleep loss are:

+ Psychological conditions such as stress, anxiety, fear, or depression.
+ Challenging bedroom environments—noisy, too hot or too cold, too bright, poor air quality, uncomfortable bed.
+ Medical and physical issues, such as breathing difficulties, pain, sickness, and hormonal issues in a woman's life.
+ Stimulants intake such as alcohol, caffeine, nicotine, drugs.
+ Overconsumption of food or liquids.
+ Circadian rhythm disruptions such as shift work, jet lag, irregular sleep habits, lengthy naps.
+ Being disturbed by a partner or child's overnight behavior.
+ Mental illnesses such as bipolar disorder and Alzheimer's disease.
+ Medically diagnosed sleep disorders (see pages 36-37).
+ Prescription medication side-effects.

# WHAT IS NATURAL SLEEP?

Natural sleep is about supporting our innate processes and presenting solutions, remedies, therapies, and techniques to heal the human body and brain without drugs, pharmaceuticals, or artificially created chemicals, to minimize risks and side effects. Respecting our natural rhythms and biological processes raises the chances of getting more consistent and lasting results over time.

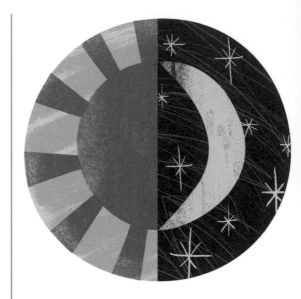

## ANCESTRAL SLEEP

A good starting point might be to learn from our ancestors, who followed a natural sleep-wake pattern and led lives centered around primal human needs, seeking protection, winding down before sleep, and following the level of light to dictate their activity and rest periods.

Sleeping like a caveman might not be entirely practical nor possible nowadays, but to be at our best we should perhaps try to bring back aspects of our original way of life and understand the disruptions we create in today's lifestyle. Mankind has not fundamentally changed constitutionally or physiologically in the last millions of years and certainly not in the last tens of thousands of years. Our brain has the same appearance and functionality.

Some scientists and academics believe that our ancestors evolved as part of a tribe, where each member played a role daytime or nighttime, which may have been passed down to us genetically, and perhaps defined our chronotype (see pages 33–34), personal attributes, and qualities.

Our sleep cycles are mostly likely a reflection of how our ancestors lived naturally as diurnal beings. In a typical day, cavemen and women would follow the darkness and light cycles, go to sleep soon after dusk in a safe, temperate haven, be active outdoors soon after dawn, and eat natural foods while fulfilling their respective tribal roles (hunter, protector, or gatherer). They might perhaps wake up a few times during the night to check for predators.

## MEDICATION AS A LAST RESORT

Resorting to sleeping pills may seem like an easy and effective way to treat sleep disorders. Although they may work for short-term sleep disruptions, unfortunately they have significant side effects not to be ignored. That is why this book presents an extensive range of non-medicated alternatives. Sleeping pills can be in the form of prescription and over-the-counter medication to be taken over a short period of time only, from a few days to a maximum of a couple of weeks, generally to treat severe insomnia due to intense periods of stress, trauma, or significant sleep disorders.

## WHAT YOU SHOULD KNOW ABOUT SLEEPING PILLS

A 2014 research study by the Associated Professional Sleep Societies found that the number of prescriptions for sleep medication in the US tripled to 20.8 million in 2010 over a 10-year period, with huge increases for non-benzodiazepine sleep medications (+350 percent), benzodiazepines (+430 percent), and other sleep medication (+200 percent).[5]

Sedative and hypnotic medication are sleep aids that impact the central nervous system (see page 22). Hypnotic sleeping pills facilitate the process of falling asleep faster or staying asleep for longer. Sedative sleeping pills create an artificial feeling of calm and cause drowsiness.

Sedative-hypnotic benzodiazepines are the most commonly prescribed sleeping pills.

Non-benzodiazepine hypnotics create less dependency than the above, but they can generate confusion and memory loss.

Antidepressants can sometimes also be used to reduce insomnia symptoms.

Some (not all) antihistamines have sedating properties.

Melatonin supplements: As explained on pages 22–23, we naturally produce the sleep hormone melatonin. Melatonin supplements are often considered a more natural and less risky option to sleeping pills, though it is unclear whether they are effective at treating insomnia consistently. They can be bought over the counter in the US (in the UK they are prescription only). Some studies have shown that taking melatonin makes it easier to fall asleep faster in primary insomnia (not linked to any other underlying medical or psychological conditions); helps regulate circadian rhythm disorders and sleep–wake patterns in blind patients; and is effective in managing jet lag when traveling or working night shifts.[6]

Not everyone agrees that melatonin should be taken to manage insomnia, except perhaps in the cases above and for the elderly. If you want to try it, it is best to take it at bedtime or a few hours before, from 0.5–5 mg depending on your sensitivity to the product. You may find that the effects wear off after a while, which is why it makes sense to explore other natural options.

Sleeping pills can unfortunately have serious side effects and may become less effective in the long term. They disrupt the naturalistic sleep–wake process and create dependency or even addiction. They can also place the patient in risky and dangerous situations. As a result, their beneficial properties may be outweighed by the negative side effects. It is always a better idea to explore natural options before taking any prescriptions. That said, all options should always be discussed with your doctor first, whether natural or pharmaceutical.

Here are some known side effects from pharmaceutical medication:

+ Dependency
+ Habit forming or addiction
+ Grogginess and sleepiness during the day
+ Memory loss
+ Confused state and lower awareness
+ Sleepwalking
+ Unusual behaviors while sleeping and not remembering when awake (eating, walking, or driving)
+ Losing balance, increasing the risk of falling, and becoming accident prone
+ Difficult rebound when stopping the medication

# KNOW THYSELF

It shouldn't be very difficult to know whether you have been sleeping enough. The signs are obvious: Good sleep generally means being in a better mood, having more energy, and being healthier in both body and mind. It is quite common, however, to tell yourself that you can get by with little sleep. A good starting point to measure your sleep is to self-monitor your daily regime and how you are feeling.

### ARE YOU SLEEPY?

Here are a few simple questions to gauge how rested you truly are:

+ Upon waking up, do you feel happy and ready for the day?
+ If you are reading during the day, could you close your eyes and fall asleep?
+ Do you often nod off, even if just for a few seconds?
+ Do you yawn frequently during the day?

---

CAUTION:  Before considering taking sleeping pills, you should consult your doctor to rule out any underlying conditions or other prescription drugs that might prevent you from sleeping soundly. Then proceed in stages to ascertain any side effects or explore natural alternatives instead. Side effects worsen if taken with even a small amount of alcohol.

- Do your eyelids feel heavy and your eyes tight and watery?
- Do you need a nap most days to feel alert and continue with your day?
- Do you easily fall asleep while commuting to and from work?
- Do you struggle staying awake or focused while in a meeting or watching TV?

If the answer is yes to some or all of these, and it is not bedtime yet, chances are that you are sleep deprived. Sleep medicine professionals routinely use an official standard questionnaire called the Epworth Sleepiness Scale (ESS) to decide whether to investigate further into potential insomnia symptoms. A medium-to-high score will suggest that you may need a polysomnography (see page 36).

## THE SLEEP DIARY: REMEMBERING YOUR DAYS AND NIGHTS

You may remember how you slept last night, but what about a week ago? Maybe not. And a month ago? It's unlikely you will remember, unless you have a regular sleep pattern or use a sleep-tracking device. This is why it is advisable to keep a sleep diary to track your nights, but also your days, to identify contributing factors to sleep. The quality of your sleep depends on what happens during your days, every step of the way. It is perhaps

more important to focus on your daytime activities than on how well you slept or not. It is quite easy to find a sleep diary template of your choice online or you can find one at www.thenaturalsleeper.com.

The best way to assess how much sleep you need is to try one of the following for a week or two:

- Allow yourself to wake up naturally— preferably with no alarm—or wake up at the same time every day (with an alarm clock or not), even at weekends.
- Go to sleep as soon as you feel sleepy at night.

While assessing your sleep needs, it is essential to:

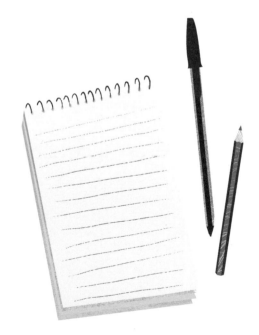

# HOW MUCH SLEEP DO YOU NEED?

*It is important not to obsess over the number of hours you sleep every night, as this isn't the only criteria to take into consideration. The recommended average is 7 to 8 hours, but we are all genetically different and some adults may feel perfectly fine with 5 hours sleep while others may need 10 to 11 hours. Our needs may also depend on our age, bearing in mind that the elderly still need pretty much as many hours as in their young adult age, but will have greater difficulty getting deep restorative sleep.*

**National Sleep Foundation's sleep duration recommendations per day:**

| | |
|---|---|
| Newborns (0–3 months) | 14–17 hours |
| Infants (4–11 months) | 12–15 hours |
| Toddlers (1–2 years) | 11–14 hours |
| Preschoolers (3–5 years) | 10–13 hours |
| School-age children (6–13 years) | 9–11 hours |
| Teenagers (14–17 years) | 8–10 hours |
| Younger adults (18–25 years) | 7–9 hours |
| Adults (26–64 years) | 7–9 hours |
| Older adults (65+ years) | 7–8 hours |

- Avoid any stimulants (activities, stimulants, drugs, or alcohol).
- Resist napping.
- Spend time outdoors daily from 20 minutes to an hour.
- Recognize signs of sleepiness—heavy eyelids, yawning, burning/dry/watery eye sensation, feeling chilly or needing to stretch—and go to sleep immediately if it is close to bedtime.
- Remember that the "second wind" we can experience after feeling very sleepy does not mean that we suddenly do not need to sleep. Instead, it is our body's stress response boosting our energy to keep going at the expense of our recovery.

Over time, your sleep-wake cycle will self-regulate, and you will wake up and fall asleep naturally at the right time for you. Remember that setting a wake-up time is most important to regulate your sleep and gauge how much sleep you need. Be aware that sleeping even just 1 or 2 hours less than what you need results in the same debilitating symptoms as having had too much alcohol (without the pleasant effects): Drowsiness, clumsiness, delayed reflexes, speech difficulties, confusion, poor judgment, and blurry vision.

## ENERGY CURVE AND CHRONOTYPES

Another way to make the most of our days and nights is to be aware of our chronotype and natural energy curve. If you can, tailor your activities and sleep to support your genetic predisposition, which dictates how your circadian rhythm behaves. Some of us might benefit more from an early night than others, who may experience better well-being from going to sleep later at night. Similarly, each person's energy curve is different, so it is important to figure out when you feel most energetic and productive during the day and target these times to accomplish intense or important activities. And rest when your energy level drops. This is also a healthy way to manage physical stress.

So, what type of sleeper are you? The general classification is:

- Extreme morning lark
- Morning lark
- Night owl
- Extreme night owl

## WHAT ABOUT PREFERENCES AND PERSONALITY TYPES?

Another approach is to be realistic about who you are, and navigate your sleep solutions based on your preferences, principles, and personality. When exploring this book, read the various options through the lenses below, or through your own lens:

+ Are you pragmatic and rational? Or more into sensory experiences and experiments?
+ Are you more "techy" and scientific? Or more into spiritual and holistic solutions?
+ Do you prefer to be assisted by a qualified professional or do you feel capable to try things on your own with minimal guidance?
+ Are you more inclined to explore mind- or body-based solutions?

## TAKING CHARGE OF YOUR SLEEP

Once you've self-monitored for a couple of weeks, and you've identified ideas you would like to try, it is time to take charge of your sleep. But first, let's reflect on the difference between being unable to sleep and not having the opportunity to get sufficient sleep.

Generally speaking, if you are unable to sleep even if you dedicate the focus, time, and care to do so, you should seek professional help. But if you are unable to sleep because you are not observing basic sleep hygiene, it will be a matter of taking control and making better lifestyle choices. Here are some thoughts on how to change this.

## ACKNOWLEDGING AND ACCEPTING HOW A LACK OF SLEEP IMPACTS YOU

Start by being honest with yourself and reflecting on what is stopping you from prioritizing supportive habits toward good sleep. What are your blockers? Are there external or psychological factors you have no control over? Those might be harder to tackle, but are you sure there isn't anything you could do about them? Or are you sticking with unhelpful patterns out of ease, comfort, pleasure, fear of change, or simply out of habit?

If this is the case, then consider how sleep deprivation impacts your life today. Could any of the following areas improve with more and better sleep? Think about your work, studies, relationships, family life, physical activity, stamina, ability to cope, or weight. And how are you feeling? Are you unhappy, depressed, unmotivated, lethargic? Wouldn't improvement in all of these areas of your life be worth the effort?

Take some time to write down on paper three incentives toward better sleep:

Not sleeping well is costing me:
My ......................................................
My ......................................................
My ......................................................

If I slept more and/or better, these are the three areas I could improve in my life today:

I could .......................................................

I could .......................................................

I could .......................................................

## COMMITTING TO CHANGE

Here are a few ideas to break old habits and form new sleep routines:

+ Choose three easy changes you feel committed to.
+ Truly understand their purpose—know the "whys."
+ Make it something you want to do, or that brings pleasure or piques your interest.
+ Stick with it: Preferably for 6 weeks but for a minimum of 3 weeks.
+ Set a realistic goal for the day
+ Signal your new habit to everyone around you, so they become your support network.
+ Don't be rigid or judgmental with yourself—be kind and supportive.
+ Be brave—face yourself without judgment or fear of what is next.
+ Be patient—don't expect overnight results (no pun intended!)

And if you are someone who has already read all the books about sleep, tried everything and given up, then step it up, make a plan, and seek professional support:

+ Get a deep dive into your psychological state of mind of the moment.
+ Enrol your doctor in analyzing any medical or physical symptoms that could prevent you from sleeping.
+ Insist on getting a polysomnography (sleep analysis) (see page 36) to uncover any potential causes.
+ Consult a specialized sleep therapist.

## BECOMING A NATURAL SLEEP EXPLORER AGAIN

*The Natural Sleeper* is designed to introduce practical and actionable solutions that are easy to understand and simple to navigate. You are your best sleep analyst and observer and are therefore invited to design your very own sleep experimentation and ritual. To find your own journey back to slumber, start by self-monitoring: Get a sense of your energetic profile, consider your preferences and personality, and understand your blockers. Then get inspired—use your instinct and gut feeling and connect with the solutions that resonate with you. What works for one person, may not work for another. This is your journey, so be curious, be brave enough to experiment, explore, and learn.

## WHEN TO SEE YOUR PRIMARY CARE PHYSICIAN

Conventional medical doctors do not consider insomnia as an illness. They see it as a by-product of another condition, which means that sleep medicine is a specialism that most primary care physicians did not study in great detail. They may not know how to identify the mundane factors that can impact your sleep, or they may think these are not medically serious enough to investigate. It is easier to work with generalist doctors as a gateway toward specialist care if you suffer from a sleep disorder that cannot be helped with any natural or alternative solution. For example, some parasomnias are serious, while others are nothing to worry too much about except if they prevent you from sleeping properly. Parasomnias provoke abnormal movements, unwanted sleep behaviors, intense emotions, and dreams, all of which can occur at any stage of sleep.

When you discuss your insomnia with your family doctor, prepare your discussion carefully:

+ Speak up about the severe impact this has on your life.
+ Prepare a list of all the sleep remedies and solutions you've already tried.
+ Prepare a list of medication you have been taking regularly.
+ Take a 2-week sleep diary with you, tracking your notes on daytime and nighttime events.

+ Be persistent about getting a sleep medicine specialist referral.
+ Insist on getting blood and thyroid tests, or any other investigative tests.
+ Request a sleep apnea test if you or your partner suspects breathing problems.
+ Request a polysomnogram (or polysomnography). This is an overnight sleep study usually conducted in a sleep clinic to diagnose sleep disorders by capturing data while you are sleeping, such as brain-wave activity, heart rate, breathing and snoring patterns, blood oxygen level, limb and eye movements. This data is captured with sensors placed on your scalp and body. Often, an observation camera is placed over the bed to observe your overnight behaviors.

There are close to 80 sleep disorders that have been identified and can be diagnosed. Here are some of the most common ones:

INSOMNIA: The most common sleep disorder, insomnia is difficulty falling or staying asleep, waking up early, and poor sleep quality, causing the patient to feel impaired and unrefreshed during the day. Someone is considered to have chronic insomnia if they have problems falling asleep or staying asleep at least three nights per week for three months or longer.

SLEEP APNEA: Interrupted breathing during sleep, whether caused by blocked passage airways or by the brain's failure to instruct the body to breathe, causes the patient to gasp for air.

RESTLESS LEG SYNDROME: An uncontrollable urge to move the legs while asleep often accompanied by a crawling sensation under the skin.

PERIODIC LIMB MOVEMENT: Repetitive, jumpy, and rhythmic movements of the leg(s) and/or arm(s) while sleeping.

CIRCADIAN RHYTHM DISORDER: Dysregulation of the body clock causing someone to go to sleep and wake up very early, or fall asleep in the morning hours and wake up late.

NARCOLEPSY: Excessive urge to fall asleep intermittently during the day.

SLEEPWALKING: Performing activities while being unaware and in an unconscious deep sleep state, not remembering behaviors and actions the next day.

REM BEHAVIOR DISORDER: When the muscular paralysis during REM phases does not occur, generating a risk as the sleeper can act out their dreams.

SLEEP PARALYSIS: Brief awakenings during REM sleep, which causes the sleeper to panic experiencing an inability to move or the perception that they cannot breathe.

HALLUCINATIONS: These can take place during the transitions between being asleep and being awake. Hypnopompic hallucinations occur as you wake up and hypnagogic hallucinations, as you fall asleep.

# REMEDIES AND THERAPIES

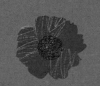

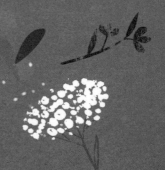

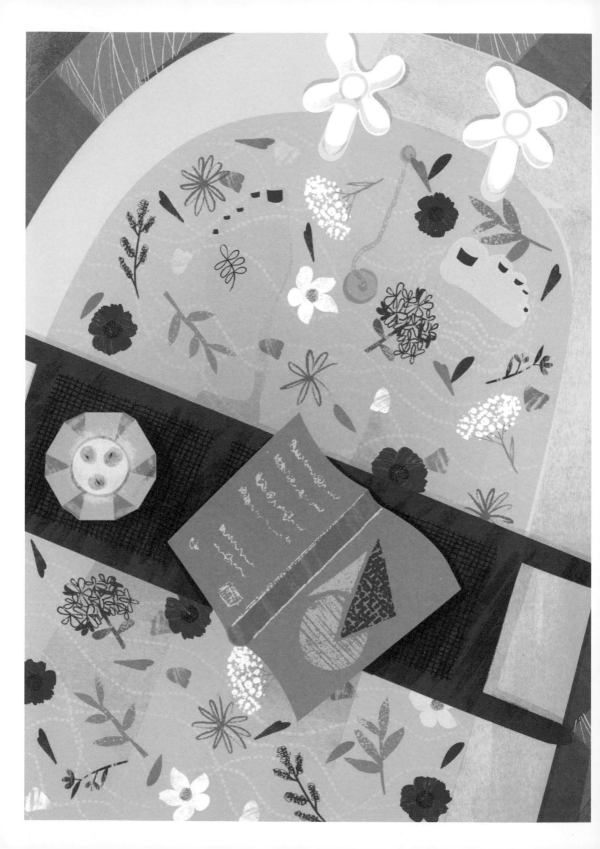

# WIND-DOWN PRACTICES AND RITUALS

Our natural physiology and behavior very much depend on our roughly 24-hour circadian rhythm, which is our natural body clock and pacemaker. To function properly, we rely on repetitive cycles at a specific rhythm. Our brain likes to know what is going to happen; it likes calculating and predicting the likely outcome of a current situation to ensure our protection, safety and, ultimately, our survival. Having a wind-down routine, or better yet a ritual, at the end of each day helps our brain and body switch from a cognitively aroused state to a relaxed state—the message is, it is okay to switch off and fall asleep. To unwind, we need to take care of the last "to dos" and process the day's memories, thoughts, and emotions so that we go to sleep with a quiet mind and relaxed body.

## THE PHYSIOLOGICAL WIND-DOWN SIGNALS

The best way to signal to the brain that it is soon time to sleep is to put signposts in place. Behavioral choices can condition your brain by subconsciously connecting these signals with sleep. You should allow for a sort of buffer before bedtime, gradually preparing both your brain and body to settle down, slowing things all the way down to doing nothing. Once the brain understands the message, it will put everything in motion with a physiological response preparing you for sleep, roughly at the same time every day. If you eliminate stress signals with a quiet mind and a relaxed body, tranquility, and darkness, then your cortisol levels will reduce further, and your parasympathetic nervous system (see page 22) will activate. Additionally, your body temperature will drop slightly, your heartbeat and blood pressure will decrease, and your breathing will naturally slow down. Meanwhile, with the right exposure to light and adequate nutrition during the day, your melatonin levels (see pages 32-34) will continue to increase, making you feel sleepy. With all the right conditions in place, you will transition blissfully into a peaceful sleep.

# A RITUAL, NOT JUST A ROUTINE

The end of each day of your life should be celebrated, reflected upon, and be seen as a chance to prepare for the next day. The aim is to make what could feel like a boring and taxing last-minute routine into a wonderful evening ritual instead.

This is an opportunity to let go of the past and prepare for the future. An opportunity to make an honest assessment of the day, reflect, manage difficult thoughts, and let go of unhelpful emotions, at least for today. It is a time to allow yourself to be calm and relaxed before sleep and remove any stress signals. The body will then anticipate and recognize your sleep ritual and cooperate.

You can get creative with your evening ritual, using however much or little time you have, but try to plan to unwind for at least 1 to 2 hours before bedtime. Your ritual should be practiced, ideally, in the following chronological order:

1. Do chores and anything else on your "to-do list" before ending your day.
2. Manage body–mind stressors, unhelpful thoughts, and emotions.
3. Plan "me" time as pressure-free self-care.
4. Welcome the morning when waking up the next day.

Think of it as the six Rs: Ritual, Relax, Rest, Repair, Recover, and then… Revive—come back anew, the next morning!

## DRAWING A LINE UNDER THE DAY

First and foremost, let's mark the end of your active day, getting the last "must dos" out of the way. These are the things you should do far in advance of bedtime, so they don't become last-minute and stressful just before sleep. The idea is to be prepared to roll into bed when the time is right, knowing you have done everything you need to. For example, household chores like washing dishes, doing laundry, or straightening the house; administrative tasks, such as paying bills or renewing subscriptions; and miscellaneous things like brushing your teeth, washing your face, preparing your clothes and lunch for the following day, locking the doors, and shutting your blinds.

## TO-DO LISTS AND PRIORITIES FOR THE FOLLOWING DAY

Then think about the "to dos" for the next day or the week ahead and prioritize them, scheduling what is urgent and important first. So that even if you have a bad night's sleep, you can still progress the A-level priority tasks and not worry about anything else. Secondly, decide what absolutely needs to be done, but can wait a little—give these tasks a B-level priority and make sure to schedule them. Finally, choose the nice-to-get-to tasks, make them a C-level priority, and schedule them for some time in the future.

This is a very important exercise, because it will take the pressure off your subconscious and conscious mind, knowing that you have prioritized what is important and when exactly you will do those tasks. This in itself sends reassuring signals to the brain, giving you permission to wind down.

## MANAGING BODY AND MIND STRESSORS

It is important to think about your evenings and identify—and then aim to reduce or eliminate—anything that could cause stress, whether small or significant. Here are a few pointers to think about:

### REDUCING STIMULATION TO YOUR SENSES

The first action should be to minimize stimulation of your physical senses, especially sight or hearing. It's a good idea to switch off electronic devices, dim down lighting around the house, and reduce the volume if you are listening to music or the radio. Also avoid consuming any stimulants before bedtime such as caffeine, cigarettes, and alcohol (see

pages 107–110). Basically avoid anything that could trick the brain into thinking it is daytime or playtime and signal it to be awake, active, and energetic.

### DOPAMINE "DETOX"

Make a point of resisting social media "addiction," binge TV viewing, playing video games, or engaging with your smartphone obsessively. You can read more about this in the Sleep Tech section, where we explain why our gadgets are so hard to ignore and why they are so addictive, and how the brain responds to a hyperconnected lifestyle (see page 177).

### MAKING PEACE BEFORE BEDTIME

Avoid conflicts at night, whether with your partner, friend, relative, or child. Aim not to go to bed angry, upset, or sad as your brain will continue processing these negative feelings and memories and store them while you sleep. Chances are this will continue to agitate you overnight even though you are sleeping, making you feel restless, resentful, or fearful, and generate a physiological stress response likely to wake you up at odd hours.

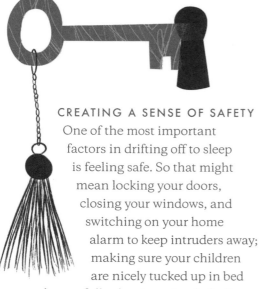

### CREATING A SENSE OF SAFETY

One of the most important factors in drifting off to sleep is feeling safe. So that might mean locking your doors, closing your windows, and switching on your home alarm to keep intruders away; making sure your children are nicely tucked up in bed and peacefully sleeping; simply feeling prepared for the next day; or hugging your partner or a nice and fluffy comfy pillow. Do whatever it takes to create a sense of safety and preparedness.

## PUTTING YOUR MIND AT EASE

An entire section of this book is called Taming the Mind (see pages 87-95), but in this segment there are more practical details about what to do before bedtime and, more specifically, how to "put the day to bed with constructive worry." Aim to do this in writing as that will help you to process the day more efficiently. If it's easier, you can use your commute time from work to carry out this exercise.

### THE GOOD AND THE "COULD BE BETTER"

Start by identifying the stresses and accomplishments of the day. Stop for a moment and reflect: What is on my mind tonight? What went well and what did not go so well? What could have been handled better, and how? Be very specific, add details, let your thoughts stream out of your mind, externalize them in writing, and channel concretely how you feel.

It is essential to consider what you can and can't control. For guidance on how best to do so, refer to the "control technique" (see pages 89-90). If you have control, then focus on one single realistic achievable thing you can do the next day. But if you don't have control, then protect your feelings by doing something supportive for yourself or someone in need, but remind yourself that it is not in your power to solve this problem. For example, if your sibling has lost their job and is in financial difficulty, research job leads for them, send them articles with financial advice, and perhaps call more often, but remember that you do not have a magic wand to make it all go away.

### YOUR SLEEP TOOLS

Being unable to sleep is often a lonely journey, so why not use one or all of the following companion tools to help you unwind, by keeping track of your sleep or bringing awareness to your feelings? These simple techniques are often used in cognitive therapy:

+ **KEEP A SLEEP JOURNAL BY YOUR BEDSIDE:** When you struggle to fall asleep or to fall back asleep after waking up in the night, or have vivid dreams or worries, grab your journal and write down whatever is going through your mind. This is a great way to diarize your feelings. Include the things that are on your mind that you need to do the next day. Write down ideas and solutions that come to you while in bed. Try to remember and interpret meaningful dreams or nightmares.

+ **EXPRESS YOUR GRATITUDE:** Thinking positively is scientifically proven to support your mental health, so write down three or more things you are grateful for each day in a dedicated notebook. Make it a habit by picking a time when you will consistently do this. Ideally, write by hand rather than digitally, so start by choosing a notebook that you love looking at and touching. In your gratitude journal include anything from small gestures to striking events or moments in your day, which simply warmed your heart and made you feel good. If you can't think of anything, look around you to find something to appreciate, think of someone you like, think about a fond memory, or something in the future you are looking forward to. Make a note of what has been good in your life, and endeavor to keep it or bring it back as often as you can.

+ **USE A "WORRY JAR":** Throw your worries, fears, and painful memories into this jar. Write each one on a piece of paper, fold it, then place it in your jar and put the lid on. Trust that your brain will do the work and find a solution in your sleep or that you are putting the worry to bed now and will deal with it the next day. Be mindful of any automatic negative thoughts (also referred to as cognitive distortions), which is when you don't see situations objectively and support negative thinking or emotions by telling yourself things that reinforce your unhelpful belief.

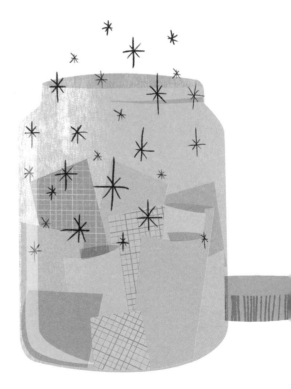

## "ME" TIME

After handling the to-dos for the evening, minimizing the stressors, reflecting on your day, and putting your mind at ease, now is the time to focus on yourself. We often sacrifice ourselves and forget to practice the self-care we need at the end of a long day. Now is the time to do something soothing, calming, restorative, regenerating, therapeutic, and healing. It is time to practice activities that are gently paced and engage the senses, but that do not cause any stress or stimulation. Also make sure to do all of these ideally outside of the bedroom.

*Note: Some of the suggestions are explained in other sections of the book, so refer to those for further details.*

- Block out some time for yourself at the end of your busy day.
- Put on your comfy nightwear and robe.
- Make a sleepy drink, such as an herbal infusion or "moon milk" at least an hour prior to sleep so you can empty your bladder before bedtime. See the Feeding Your Sleep (page 102) and Healing Plants (page 160) sections for inspiration for sleepy drinks.
- Do something pleasant like easy reading, watching your favorite comedy show, listening to light music, or catching up casually with your friends on the phone.
- Practice your favorite relaxing hobby, such as drawing, singing, painting, or knitting.
- Practice gentle exercise such as yoga nidra poses (see page 75) or Qigong (see page 100) to release tension and pain in the body before bed, readjust back alignment, and keep the muscles flexible, strong, and healthy.
- Engage in other sensory activities such as getting a massage, intimacy with someone, lighting an aromatherapy candle, or switching on your aromatherapy diffuser with drops of a relaxing essential oil (see pages 170–175).
- If you still don't feel sleepy, practice techniques likely to activate your parasympathetic nervous system and feel relaxed such as controlled breathing (see pages 76–77) or meditation techniques (see page 78).

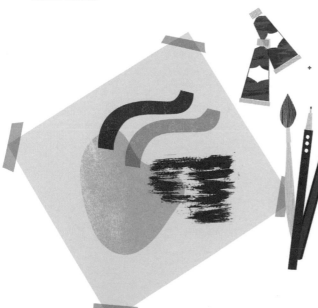

+ You may choose to pray or chant mantras to lift or appease your soul and spirit.

## SLEEPING BEAUTY

One way to wind down and feel great inside and out is to engage in a pre-bedtime beauty ritual, and prepare for the natural skin repair process that takes place while we sleep. Beauty sleep is a natural matter as scientifically proven by the Swedish Karolinska Institute. Their study found that "sleep-deprived people appeared less healthy and less attractive than after a normal night's sleep" according to a survey panel[1]. Being tired often means looking pale and having swollen or red eyes, dry skin, and dark circles under the eyes. Our low energy is conveyed through our facial expressions, which may not be socially engaging nor attractive. The National Sleep Foundation states that cleansing and moisturizing your skin before sleep gives better results, reducing breakouts and dehydration and helps prevent wrinkles[2].

## YOUR BATH OR SHOWER RITUAL

The thought of soaking in hot and steamy water at the end of a day sounds divine doesn't it? So why not make it a sleep ritual? In addition to releasing tension and being pleasurable, it raises then later on lowers the body temperature, which in itself induces sleep quite magically. Cooling the body down is one of the physiological signals indicating that it is time to sleep. Science experts suggest doing so 1.5 to 2 hours before bedtime for a maximum effect.

## WELCOMING THE DAY

Whatever your sleep was like during the night, and however refreshed you may feel, make sure to celebrate the start of a new day and get ready for your morning ritual. Rather than letting an alarm clock startle you out of sleep, and instead of immediately diving into your social media feed, prepare yourself for the day as follows:

+ Wake up at the same time every day, even at weekends. Ideally wake up with the daylight rather than an alarm, but if you do use an alarm try not to snooze it.
+ Let natural light in as close to wake-up time as possible to help reduce any sensations of inertia—stand by your open window or go outside.
+ Give yourself time to wake up with a gentle gradual rise rather than jumping out of bed. Start with a moment of peace.
+ Awaken your senses by breathing in, put your feet up against the wall while laying down to increase blood circulation to your heart and brain; sit up and roll your shoulders and neck; massage your entire face and scalp in circular motions; do some stretches.
+ Then think about the day ahead and the A-level (see pages 42–43) priorities you will focus on for the day.

## CREATING YOUR OWN DAILY SLEEP RITUAL

*Use this chart to jot down ideas you've selected when reading this book to create your personalized sleep ritual. Place each chosen element of your ritual in the order you prefer and a time of day you will commit to doing it.*

**My daily steps to prepare for sleep**

1 ...........................................................
2 ...........................................................
3 ...........................................................
4 ...........................................................
5 ...........................................................
6 ...........................................................
7 ...........................................................

**Time of day**

1 ...........................................................
2 ...........................................................
3 ...........................................................
4 ...........................................................
5 ...........................................................
6 ...........................................................
7 ...........................................................

# ABOUT NAPPING

Napping or having a little siesta is a daily wind-down ritual in many cultures and, of course, a must for young children. While naps have been proven to be beneficial for the brain, they can disrupt our sleep-wake cycles, so it is best to nap responsibly.

Naps are necessary in extreme circumstances, for certain sleep disorders, and for specific professions requiring focus, high precision, and concentration at all times, such as drivers, pilots, surgeons, night-workers, ER staff, military people, firefighters, and construction workers, to avoid accidents and mistakes. Parents of young children might also need naps to be able to function after a night of disrupted sleep.

Naps are good for concentration, performance, alertness, vigilance, transferring recent memories into our long-term memory, to strengthen our immune system, for hormonal regulation, to cope with stress, for good mood, and healthy blood pressure, and to reduce sensitivity to pain.

That said, napping is generally not advised for chronic insomniacs or the elderly because it reduces the buildup of sleep pressure and feeds into the vicious cycle of insomnia. If your inability to sleep is severe, then the only type of "nap" recommended is a micro-nap (micro-sleep) whereby you are allowed to rest without properly sleeping. This can be done anywhere—at your desk, on public transport, in a waiting room. Simply close your eyes, resting from a few seconds to 5 minutes at the most.

Feeling sleepy and craving for a nap after lunchtime is normal and not related to digesting your food. It is called the post-lunch circadian dip, which takes place between 1–3:30 pm whether you ate or not, right when daylight starts decreasing, which is generally 6 to 7 hours after waking up, at which point our vigilance and attention decrease.

If you really need it and if your sleep debt is not too high, you can take a short nap but not too late in the day:

+ Your power nap should not last more than 30 minutes (ideally 15 to 20 minutes)—set an alarm to make sure you don't sleep for too long. You will enter stage 1 or 2 light sleep, which will be easy to wake up from and shouldn't affect your sleep drive.
+ Don't nap later than 7 hours before bedtime, i.e. roughly no later than 4 pm.
+ Remember, napping has lots of benefits and it helps support sleep deprivation, but it does not replace nocturnal sleep.

Alternatively, to resist napping:

+ Take a 5–10 minute pause every 90–120 minutes, stretch, get up, go outside, and breathe deeply.
+ Alternate doing manual and intellectual activities.
+ Meditate, practice mindfulness, or do something mindless, requiring no intention to do or think about something. Allow autopilot to take over by, for example, going for a walk, looking at the sky out of the window, doing some cleaning or ironing, massaging your neck, stretching.

## DEALING WITH NOCTURNAL AWAKENINGS

There are many reasons why we may wake up in the middle of the night and you are best placed to self-monitor and understand your sleep patterns. But, broadly speaking, any excessive physical or mental stimulation or any disturbances to the naturalistic physiological sleep–wake process will disrupt our sleep.

Once you've read through this book, you will have a better understanding of what is happening and you can then come back to this section with a clearer idea of what to do next. If you wake up during the night and can't fall back asleep, go through the following mental checklist and act as fast as possible so you can quickly find your way back to sleep:

+ **DO I NEED TO EMPTY MY BLADDER?** If so, go to the bathroom immediately. The longer you wait, the more difficult it will be to fall back asleep because your alertness will have increased.

+ **AM I THIRSTY AND DEHYDRATED?** Some people experience night awakening or anxiety because they are dehydrated while they are sleeping, and the body goes in full alert until it feels hydrated again. Take sips of water, rather than gulping down a full glass to avoid frequent bathroom runs later in the night.

+ **DID I DRINK ALCOHOL OR HAVE CAFFEINE YESTERDAY?** If so, drink water (even if this might wake you later on) and open a window for fresh air, but the best advice is to avoid or limit consumption hours before sleep.

+ **AM I TOO HOT?** If so, uncover, remove blanket layers, or open a window. Consider using a fan, a cool pack, or air-conditioning during heatwaves. Review the Building your Cocoon (page 53) and Sleep Tech (page 177) sections for further information on ways to help with feeling hot in bed.

+ **AM I TOO COLD?** If so layer up and prepare a hot-water bottle, which will later cool down and therefore induce sleep more effectively than an electric blanket. See pages 55–56 for pointers on the ideal temperature to sleep.

+ **AM I ANXIOUS?** Is my heart racing? If something stressful is on your mind refer to the Beditation (page 75), Taming the Mind (page 87), or Sound Asleep (page 149) sections for practical calming techniques, including controlled breathing and journaling, which are very efficient ways to fall back asleep.

+ **AM I EXCITED?** If so, grab your sleep journal and write freely to celebrate or prepare for a great event ahead.

+ **IS IT NOISY?** If so, reduce or mask disturbing noises as much as you can— refer to the Sound Asleep section for some ideas. If the noise disturbance comes from your bed partner, you may want to consider moving to another room.

+ **IS THERE ANY SOURCE OF LIGHT IN MY BEDROOM AT ALL, EVEN IF VERY FAINT?** If so, block or cover it up and ensure complete darkness. If you need to get up in the night, use dim lighting or a torch light to move around. If you are afraid of the dark, explore cognitive behavioral therapy (CBT—see pages 88-89), increase your exposure to the dark gradually until you feel safe, and practice controlled breathing techniques (see pages 76-77).

◆ **DO I HAVE ANY PAINS OR A HEADACHE?** If so try to relieve your pain immediately, whether naturally or by taking pain medication if all else fails. Try using a satin bed-sliding sheet on top of your regular bed sheet if you experience back or hip pain, are pregnant, have arthritis, or mobility restrictions while in bed. This tubular piece of fabric is slippery on the inside, which will faciliate your movements in bed and with changing sides as you toss and turn.

◆ **COULD I BE LOW IN BLOOD SUGAR?** Hunger or low blood sugar can cause you to wake up. Avoid this by eating a light protein-rich snack ahead of bedtime.

◆ **AM I JET-LAGGED?** If so, see the jet lag advice on pages 71–73.

If you are still unable to fall back asleep after 15 to 20 minutes, leave your bedroom and sit down in another dimly lit or dark room, with no stimulation of any kind. Stay there until you start feeling slightly chilly, as this will help you to nod off faster. As soon as your eyes start to sting, and feel heavy and dry, ready to close, or if you start yawning, go to bed immediately and let yourself drift off to sleep.

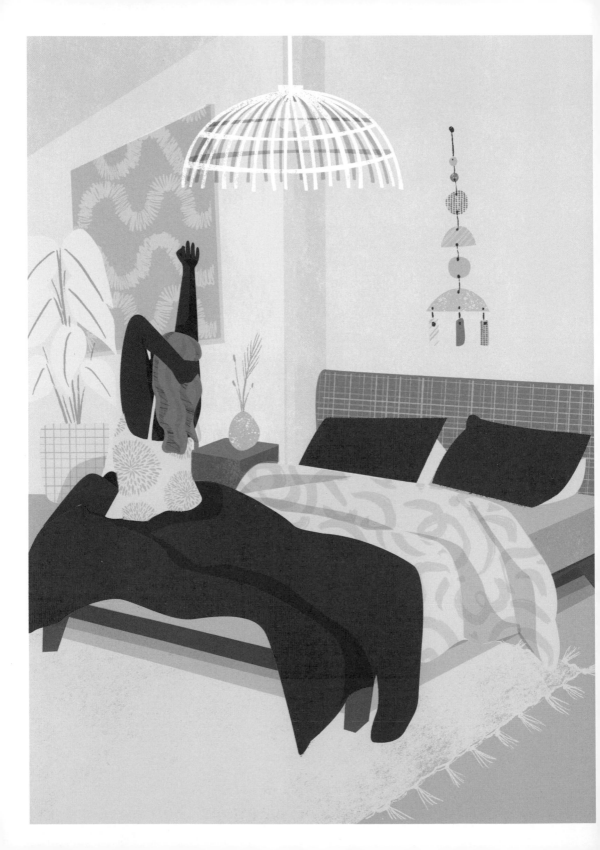

# BUILDING YOUR COCOON

When it came to sleeping, our ancestors were particular about finding a perfect spot and creating an ideal environment, and that's probably why our sleeping arrangements and surroundings are such an important part of getting a good night's sleep. In this section, you will learn why it is essential to create a bedroom setting and ambience that makes you feel safe and comfortable—a space that is quiet, cool, and dark—and discover how to make your bedroom your very own comforting and protective cocoon, your restorative sanctuary, and peaceful haven.

## MIGHTY TIDY

The first step in creating the right ambience is to remove clutter from your bedroom and any objects related to wakeful activities. So that means no electronics, no tablets, no game console, and definitely no television or computers. The idea is for your bedroom to become an area where you detox from any connected or stimulating devices, with the possible exception of a small alarm clock (it is better to use this than your phone as an alarm), an aromatherapy diffuser (see page 173), a fan, and a humidifier, if needed. If you suffer from chronic insomnia (see page 36), it is best not to have any books or magazines in the bedroom either.

## SLEEP—NOTHING ELSE

There are many things you may want to use your bedroom for, but you should dedicate this cocoon solely to sleep and sexual activity. This advice is backed by sleep medicine professionals and psychologists alike, supported by cognitive behavioral therapy for insomnia (CBTi; see pages 88-89), and feng shui philosophy (see page 54): The bedroom should be a place for rest and intimacy only. Nothing else. It is important to create and maintain a subconscious association between your sleep and your bedroom, which should not be used as your office, library, or living room.

If you suffer from chronic insomnia, it is not recommended to read, take phone calls, or text chat in bed either. Bedtime should not be used to catch up on your work emails or social media feeds. At the most, your bedroom can be the place where you get dressed, but ideally for no longer than 15-20 minutes. If you live in a studio and have no choice but to have wakeful activity near where you sleep, then make sure to place any items related to this as far away from the bed as possible—for example, use a room divider, screen, curtain, or plant to create a separation.

## ENERGY FLOW AND AMBIENCE

To structure your bedroom for sleep and peace, how about following some of the feng shui principles to create a harmonious feel? Feng shui (pronounced "fung shway") is an ancient Chinese interior design discipline and philosophy guiding you on how to set up your home and surroundings in harmony and balance, to generate a powerful energy flow throughout your home leading to happiness, success, good relationships, health, wealth, and protection. This energy should flow without any obstructions, sharp angles, or reflecting objects like mirrors. Feng shui tips for the bedroom include:

+ Position your bed against a solid wall, facing toward the door but not right in front of it.
+ Avoid any underbed storage that would create heavy or stagnant energy underneath you.
+ The atmosphere should feel soothing, relaxing, and calming, with neutral colors and decorations that make you feel good and positive.
+ It is a good idea to balance materials and textures in your bedroom, such as wood, metal, stone, fabric, and glass.

## DIM DOWN, THEN PITCH DARK

To wind down, your evening lighting should reduce progressively, just like the sunset. Choose lighting that can be dimmed down, all the way to complete darkness. You have a choice of ceiling lights with dimmers, low-light bedside lamps, sunset simulator lamps, or a simple Himalayan salt lamp to create soothing bedroom lighting.

Limit, reduce, or avoid exposure to blue light (see pages 66–67) or any light coming from electronic devices, electric chargers, indicator lights, and alarm clocks. Cover, hide, or turn them away from your eyesight, however faint they might be. You might otherwise not release sufficient melatonin (see page

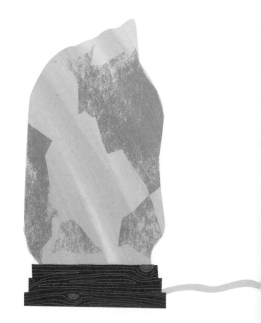

22) to stay asleep because it is not totally pitch dark. Even the slightest light levels can be perceived through your eyelids when closed. Install blackout curtains or blinds to block out any exterior night-lights or to avoid being woken up by (too) early morning sunrays. As a backup a light-blocking eye mask can do the trick, especially at sunrise, which can start very early. Ideally, though, if you follow natural sleep–wake cycles, you would go to sleep soon after sunset and wake up with the sunrise, in which case you would not need an alarm clock, blackout curtains, or eye masks.

## SHHHH... SILENCE PLEASE

Quietness is absolutely essential for a good night's sleep. Our hearing sense stays alert at all times, even while we are in our deepest sleep. This is likely linked to our ancestors needing to protect themselves from dangerous predators at night. They needed to differentiate unusual noises indicating a potential danger or a threat requiring their attention at any time, especially when asleep, one of their most vulnerable moments. So avoid being jerked out of sleep and make sure that unusual noises don't prevent you from entering deep sleep. Should you not be able to avoid environmental noise, then read the Healing Sounds section on page 150 for ideas on how to cover it up. Other

options to protect yourself from startling external noises might be to install double-glazed windows, which provide sound insulation, or think about sound-insulating your whole bedroom if needed. If the noise comes from your bed partner, then you may want to consider wearing foam or silicon earplugs. Allow foam earplugs to adjust after inserting them in the ear openings; silicon earplugs need to be molded with your fingers, then placed and fitted in the opening. Or else maybe choose to sleep in a separate room, although, of course, this may not be an easy choice. See pages 61–62 for further suggestions on peaceful sleep, alone (or not).

## THE RIGHT TEMPERATURE

If your core body temperature is elevated and you feel warm or hot, there is a good chance you will struggle to fall or stay asleep. The same goes for if you feel too cold. An inadequate environmental temperature will most likely disrupt REM sleep. With thermoregulation, our internal body temperature naturally fluctuates by 2–3°F degrees throughout the day and night, and decreases slightly at bedtime which helps us fall asleep, then rises equally upon waking up. The average person's lowest body temperature is generally lowest about two hours before wake up time—around 5 am on average. The brain and body's temperature also lowers during NREM sleep. This is all part of our sleep-wake process. Therefore, you should aim to keep your bedroom cool at 60–67°F. Young children and elderly people may require a slightly warmer environment. If you feel chilly easily, then you can place a hot-water bottle or a heated electric blanket in the bed before slipping into your sheets, but make sure that you remove it or turn it off as you lay down. Be mindful that it should never be any hotter than 84°F underneath the covers.

To achieve a comfortable temperature in your bed, you may also want to consider the bedding materials and mattress you sleep on—refer to pages 186–187 for guidance on temperature-controlled (also called thermo-regulated) fabrics and materials. You may also want to look into "smart" mattresses that adjust the temperature under the covers for a more comfortable sleep (see page 187).

Your body heat is regulated through the skin surface while you are sleeping, so it is a good idea to keep your face, head (scalp), hands, and feet either in the open air or covered, as needed.

Besides adjusting your room and bed temperature, be mindful of anything you might have ingested throughout the day that could increase your body temperature such as alcoholic, sugary, and caffeinated drinks.

## OPTIMAL AIR QUALITY

A well-ventilated and oxygenated bedroom is very important to improve sleep quality[1]. Consider opening your windows and doors before going to bed to allow fresh air to flow into your room. This will reduce the levels of carbon dioxide and potentially reduce the bedroom temperature, and it will help you to breathe and give you a sense of well-being immediately. You should also pay attention to the humidity levels and use a humidifier or dehumidifier to make sure the air is neither too dry nor too damp. Either can affect your breathing. Waking up with a dry mouth, lips, or skin, or having nosebleeds during the night, are signs that the air is too dry.

# FEELING SAFE

Never underestimate the need to feel safe before going to sleep. Safety from physical or psychological dangers is an absolute requirement to sleep, so remove any perceived danger from your home and bedroom. Our ancestors were seemingly seeking refuge inside dark caverns to stay protected from predators and find the peace, quietness, and shelter needed for sleep. Interpret this however you'd like for yourself, whether it is making sure your front door is locked, windows closed, home alarm switched on, hugging your pillow, or snuggling with your partner. If you feel unsafe and cannot resolve this on your own, seek help and support. Perhaps also read the Taming the Mind section of this book (see pages 87-95) and explore some mind management techniques to help manage anxieties and worries.

# A COMFORTABLE AND COMFORTING BED

Once your bedroom environment is sorted out, it is time to pay respect and attention to perhaps the most important material piece of the sleep puzzle—your bed. You will spend on average about one-third of your life in bed, so that's approximately 248,200 hours, assuming a life expectancy of 85 years. Choose your bed carefully and do not hesitate to invest in quality and durability.

When you purchase a bed, you should acquire the mattress and the bed base at the same time and make sure that one doesn't counteract the properties of the other. The bed base, or bed frame, is equally important in absorbing impact and weight. If chosen properly, it will protect the mattress and prevent it from slumping too quickly, while ensuring good ventilation, both of which will help the mattress last for longer and stay in a better and more hygienic condition. Bed bases are generally solid divan or slatted, with rigid or flexible slats.

When purchasing a bed and mattress, definitely try before you buy to ensure the appropriate comfort and support. Do take your time and spend at least 10 minutes lying on the bed and mattress in the store before deciding which one is right for you. Ignore anyone giving you an amused look while you test beds for a while—this is an important investment! You will find a good overview here, but as always be guided by your own personal preferences and seek further professional advice if necessary. It is advisable to look at non-commercial online sources for unbiased pointers and advice.

## YOUR MATTRESS

It is time to change your mattress when you notice bumps or holes, if you start to roll in against your bed partner (if you have one), if the mattress doesn't come back into its original shape after a little while, if it is dirty or smelly, or if you feel stiffness, aches, and pains when you wake up. Each adult releases typically half a liter of perspiration every night on average, sometimes more, a lot of which ends up in the mattress. It is generally advised to change your mattress every 7 years, so this means you are investing for approximately 20,440 hours of sleep over 2,555 days.

Ensure that you purchase a large enough mattress for two people if you sleep with a partner. You might want to consider having separate mattresses linked by a zipper, so each of you can choose different mattress tensions if needed or to avoid being disturbed by each other's movements.

The key to sleep comfort is to choose a mattress that provides good spine alignment when you lie down in whichever position. Therefore you should choose a mattress tension that is neither too firm nor too soft for you, preferably one that is available on a trial basis. The options are usually soft, medium, firm, or extra firm. Generally speaking, light-weighted people should avoid firm mattresses, and heavier individuals should avoid soft tension, as it creates unnecessary muscle stiffness overnight.

Your body shape matters, too—people with wide hips or curved bodies should opt for medium to soft mattresses, allowing the hips to sink enough into the mattress for the spine to be aligned. You may want to consider body-responsive mattresses that simplify the choice.

There are several types of mattress that fall either under the "with springs" (sprung) and the "without springs" (non-sprung) categories. There are also hybrids with both categories, for example springs and foam combined.

When it comes to spring interior mattresses, pocket sprung or open sprung are the most popular mattresses. The more springs they contain, the more support, ventilation, and bounce they can offer. These mattresses are recommended for heavier or single people, and for those who sweat a lot at night. Manufacturers can customize and adjust the mattress firmness by zone, giving more support for desired parts of the body. Interior sprung mattresses can be made with a wide range of fillings such as cotton, wool, foam, polyester, silk, cashmere, natural fiber, and horsehair.

There are four main types of non-sprung mattresses: Gel, floatation, futons, and foam.

+ **GEL** is a relatively recent filling that provides breathability, pressure relief, and body support.
+ **FLOATATION** means water- or liquid-filled, and provides pressure-free

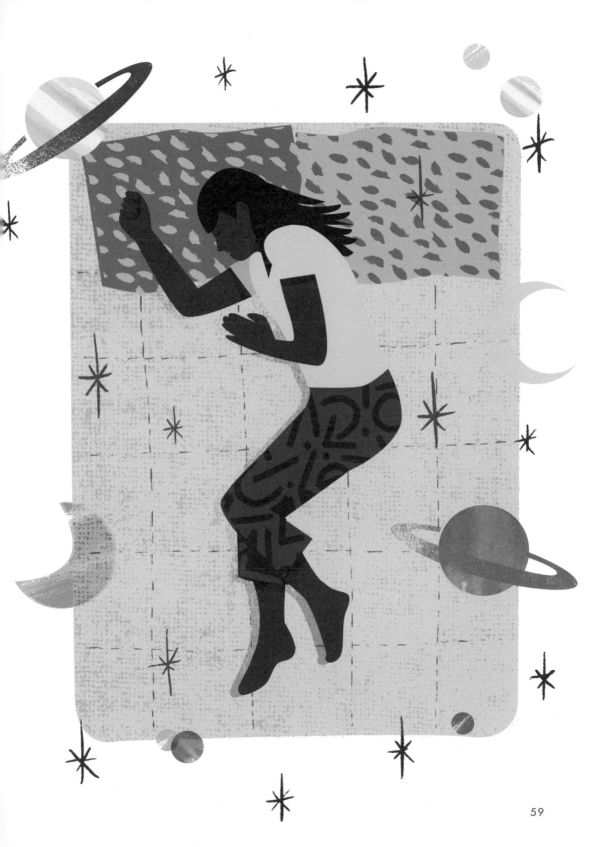

support and is appropriate for allergy sufferers.

+ **FUTONS**, originally from Japan, are used on the floor or on a slatted frame and are made with cotton and a fiber-filling material.

There are three main types of foam mattress: Latex, memory foam, and polyurethane foam.

+ **LATEX** is a more expensive option, but it is comfortable, breathable, and provides better support and more durability. It is available in synthetic or natural material; the latter being less likely to make you sweat.
+ **MEMORY FOAM** is more affordable but not as durable. It gives firm support and is responsive to the shape of your body, but can make some people overheat. The denser it is, the easier it goes back to its initial shape.
+ **POLYURETHANE FOAM** is a variation that seems to be body-temperature sensitive and can cause sweating.

A few words about mattress maintenance:

+ Avoid bending or rolling a sprung mattress as this will damage it.
+ Make sure to ventilate your mattress regularly, ideally by standing it upward.
+ Air the room and vacuum the mattress regularly to minimize dust and dust mites.

+ Turn it and rotate it regularly, except if it is the non-turn kind, especially in the first few months, to prolong its life span.

## YOUR BEDDING

Your sleep experience wouldn't be complete without good bedding. Again, it is worth the investment in quality. You may want to consider breathable and thermo-regulated sleepwear and bedding (see page 186), or opt for natural materials and fabrics such as cotton and linen, which are perhaps more cooling and comfortable. Avoid covering up with multiple blankets on the bed, especially during hot months as it may become uncomfortable.

### PILLOWS

Make sure that your neck is supported by an appropriate pillow. The key is to select one that is neither too thin, nor too thick to ensure correct spine-neck alignment. The pillow should shape around the neck and support the head. There is a wide choice of pillows available, and the main categories are:

+ Standard pillows made of either polyester, feather, down, microfiber, or memory foam.
+ Wool or latex foam pillows.
+ Specialist and ergonomic pillows to alleviate allergies, snoring, and cervical neck pain.

### WEIGHTED SLEEP PRODUCTS

- Eye pillows are simple cases filled with beads or flaxseeds to be rested on your closed eyes, for a moment of relaxation and acupressure around the eyes. Sometimes infused with aromatic oils or dried herbs, eye pillows are meant to help relieve headaches, insomnia, and eye strain.

- Weighted blankets are reported to help release serotonin, oxytocin, and dopamine and keep your nervous system calm by simulating the feeling of being held. Their properties are based on stimulation and acupressure principles, by distributing the weight and pressure evenly across your body while keeping you at the right temperature. Weighted blankets are said to reduce nighttime anxieties, stress, and insomnia by helping reduce levels of the stress hormone cortisol.

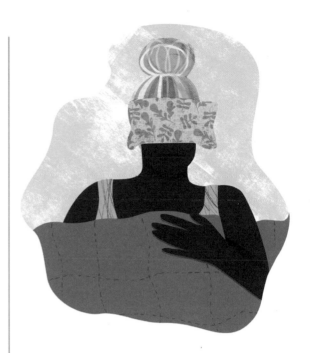

## PEACEFUL SLEEP, ALONE...OR NOT

Sharing a bed with someone is one thing, but doing so comfortably is another. It is a matter of negotiation as we each have our favorite sleep preferences, such as the preferred time to go to sleep, ideal mattress tension, preferred side of the bed, preferred position, and room temperature. And then we can disturb each other with overnight tossing and turning, snoring, bathroom runs, light on or off . . . there are many legitimate reasons why you might decide to sleep apart, and that's okay. Or, of course, you can concede . . . as long as you don't compromise too much on your sleep. A compromise might be to sleep in side-by-side mattresses or in separate twin beds. Otherwise, choosing to sleep in separate beds and bedrooms may mean more sleep for each of you, and therefore better mood, better sex, and better sociability with each other. Whereas a lack of sleep can lead to moody behavior, irritability, and destructive arguments.

There is, however, scientific evidence as to why it feels good to co-sleep. The closeness with a bed partner triggers a release of oxytocin often called the "love" or "pleasure" hormone, giving a relaxing and sleep-inducing response, and a sense of feeling safe and protected. Co-sleeping

## FURRY FRIENDS

Sleeping with a pet in your bed is a matter of preference and hygiene principles, but it is generally not recommended if the presence of your favorite animal companion disrupts your sleep due to additional noise and movements, or if their body temperature makes you feel too warm. This might also be a point of negotiation if your partner objects to having a pet in the bed. Research found that 13 percent of surveyed couples disagree about whether a dog should sleep in the bed with them or not.[2] One solution might be to explore bedside pet beds, which can be on the ground or elevated at mattress level.

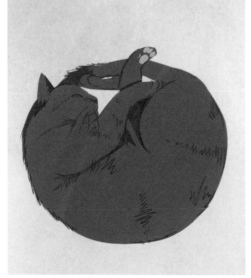

with babies and children is controversial because of safety concerns and the impact on their psychology, although it feels quite natural for babies and toddlers to sleep on or very near their mother's body. Communal sleeping as a family in preindustrial times was the norm because of poverty and lack of heating. Beds were expensive and communal sleeping with all family members and household animals was the standard for poorer families, while the rich would sleep in separate beds and rooms.

# ALTERNATIVE BEDROOMS AND ACCESSORIES

Here are a few other ideas to soothe your spirit and perhaps improve your sleep.

### DREAM CATCHERS

Originally made by indigenous people of the Americas, dream catchers are protective objects hung over the beds of babies and children. They are meant to deflect and protect them from bad dreams and evil spirits. You may be familiar with these round hoops and woven nets made of yarn, then decorated with beads and feathers. They represent good energy and may help to neutralize bad energy. Consider finding an indigenous maker if you'd like to purchase a dreamcatcher.

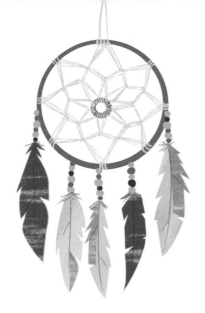

experience that makes us feel at one with the universe and enhances our connection to nature. It is worth experimenting with such a concept for your next summer vacation, whether in an open-air camping or glamping site, in a transparent glass igloo, in a panoramic tent, or in a yurt or treehouse. Why not try it? Just ensure that you keep yourself at the right temperature.

## HAMMOCKS

Supporters of hammocks believe that they are more comfortable than mattresses and put you in an ideal position for good sleep. Swaying back and forth in a hammock may make you feel relaxed and happy, helping you to fall asleep faster and sleep more deeply. A common explanation is that hammocks are associated with relaxation, stress-free vacations, and perhaps a laid-back lifestyle, yet scientific studies[3] in mice and humans showed that rocking back and forth may actually "synchronize" brain waves in a way that promotes deeper sleep, and may increase stage 2 non-REM sleep and improve sleep quality and memory.

## STARGAZING

Falling asleep under a starry sky might be the most natural and extraordinary setting for a bedroom—a humbling

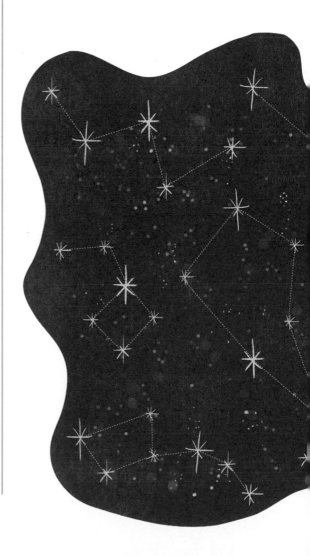

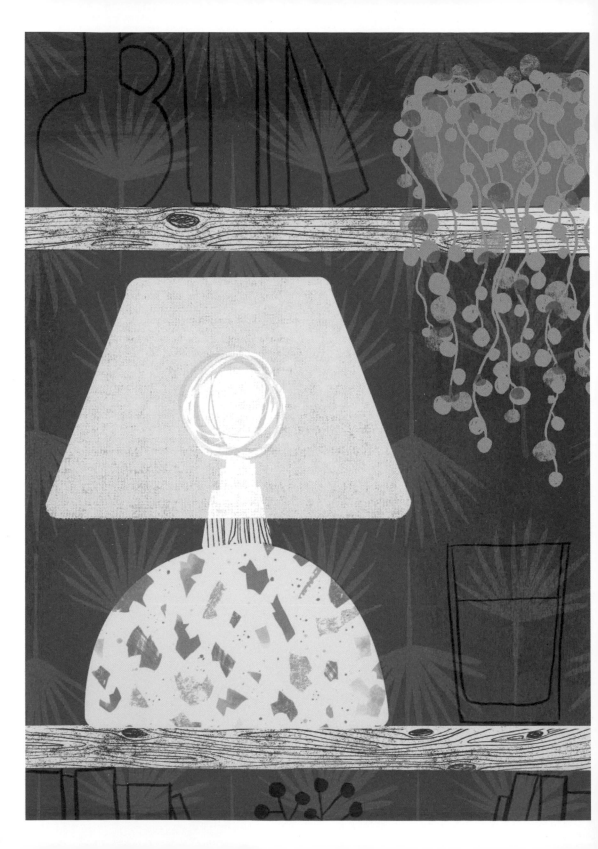

# SEEING THE LIGHT

Our exposure to light, more specifically sunlight, is possibly the most important influencing factor in getting a good night's sleep. The level of light is the primary "zeitgeber," sending a signal to our brain that it is time to either wake up or go to sleep. A zeitgeber is a physiological marker that acts as a cue in the regulation of the body's circadian rhythm (body clock). So let's first understand how light impacts our sleep-wake cycle, then find out when it can be our ally, or sometimes our enemy, when it comes to sleep.

## LET THERE BE LIGHT

As nature intended, our sleep-wake cycle follows a regular repetitive pattern, alternating between sleep and wakefulness on a daily basis. This is the result of changes in neurotransmitters and hormones as a response to our exposure to the 24-hour darkness/daylight cycle. Two processes are working together: Our internal master clock, also called the circadian rhythm or body clock, and our sleep drive, also called sleep pressure. These two allies join forces to help us fall asleep and wake up within a 24-hour period on average (anywhere between 23h30 and 24h30).

+ Sleep pressure determines how sleepy we feel, and it builds up thanks to a neurotransmitter in the brain called adenosine, which increases gradually throughout the day and makes us feel sleepy by the end of the day, as the hours go by. Then, adenosine levels decrease during sleep.

+ Our circadian rhythm determines when we should be asleep. The body clock is regulated by synchronizing with the rise and fall of natural light levels, which signal to our brain when to be awake, alert, and active, and when to fall asleep.

So how does it work? Certain photosensitive cells in our eyes measure light brightness and perceive the visible wavelength that corresponds to a specific color of the light spectrum. These photoreceptors signal nightfall and daylight to a part of our brain called the suprachiasmatic nucleus (SCN) located right behind our eyes within the hypothalamus. Our eye sensors are more sensitive to detecting blue light, which is a shorter wavelength than other colors in the natural daylight spectrum. When our SCN perceives both the color and brightness of the light, it orders our brain to release or suppress the sleep hormone melatonin, which in turn helps regulate our internal master clock.

## SUNSET

When the sun lowers and it gets darker outside, the SCN signals the pineal gland at the base of our brain to release the hormone melatonin, which has a sedative effect and makes us fall asleep. Melatonin is released throughout the night to keep us asleep, peaking at around 3 am, then gradually decreasing to its lowest level right before dawn, when it is wake-up time.

## SUNRISE

When the sun rises, the same eye sensors exposed to the morning's more intense blue light send the signal to our SCN to halt the release of the sleep hormone melatonin to help us feel more awake and alert. It is blue light, in particular, that tells the master clock that it is the beginning of daytime. It synchronizes itself with the start of the day and prompts us to feel alert. Blue light is on the cooler end of the visible light spectrum and is generated naturally by the sun, although it can also be emitted by screens from artificial lighting and electronic device screens.

## WHAT ABOUT ARTIFICIAL LIGHT?

The invention of electric lighting and screen-based electronic devices has been such a revolutionary phenomenon bringing ease and comfort into our homes. The trouble is that artificial lighting has undoubtedly been disrupting our sleep both because of the extended exposure to it and because of the lifestyle changes it caused. We use artificial lighting in the evening for activities we would otherwise not do, which delays both our bedtime and the release of melatonin, which in turn delays our sleep onset (when we fall asleep), leading to a shorter night's sleep.

We often stare into light-emitting screens for hours before bedtime and engage in active, wakeful, or stressful activities on these devices, which confuses the brain as to what time it is and inhibits our natural desire to sleep.

## BLUE LIGHT AND LED LIGHTS

Sunlight and white light contain a mixture of wavelengths, colors, and a fair amount of blue light. Undimmed LED (light-emitting diode) lighting and electronic device screens are known to release more blue light than other light sources, such as fluorescent and incandescent bulbs. Whether walking up LED-lit streets at night, lighting up our living rooms with racks of bright

LED ceiling spotlights, or by actively engaging in our smartphones, TVs, tablets, computers, or even e-readers in the hours before bedtime, we expose ourselves to probably more artificial light than we should, right up until we crash in bed. During the night, even the slightest light coming from an alarm clock display could disrupt our sleep. Blue light in the evening fools our brain into thinking it is still daytime, which is known to suppress the natural release of melatonin.

### THE BLUE LIGHT DEBATE

A scientific study also shows that it isn't just blue color but also bright yellow color that can impact the circadian rhythm.[1] In addition to this, research found that is not only the color but also the brightness that can impact our sleep quantity and quality.[2] So if you increase the brightness of your screen to improve readability, this will counterbalance the benefit of blue light filter products such as apps or eyeglasses.

A perhaps contradicting study says that blue light may not be as detrimental to sleep as assumed. Scientists found that exposure to blue light from an e-reader did suppress the release of melatonin, but it had a modest impact on sleep: fewer than 10 minutes longer to fall asleep and under 10 minutes less REM sleep, compared to those reading a print book, and there was no impact on total sleep duration or deep sleep.[3]

What seems reasonable for everyone, however, is that exposure to blue light during the day, whether natural or artificial, should not influence our sleep patterns.

## THE IDEAL DAILY "LIGHTS ROUTINE"

As you read previously, light is your friend when it comes to sleep, especially if it is used in the most natural fashion. Here are some pointers on how to follow an ideal lights routine, to feel sleepy at bedtime and alert in the daytime:

### DAYTIME

+ Wake up at the same time every single day, including at weekends.
+ Get some natural light exposure outdoors early morning, as soon as possible after waking up: Look out

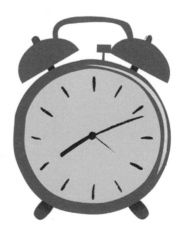

from your opened window, enjoy your garden or balcony, go for a run.

+ Get as much natural sunlight as you can during the day by being outdoors, rain or shine—no less than 30 minutes, ideally between the hours of 10 am and 3 pm in winter and between 9 am and 5 pm in summer. Even a brief lunchtime walk can make a difference. Of course, don't forget to apply your sunblock to avoid sunburn.

+ Exercise outdoors in the daylight.

+ Feel free to lie down in the grass or on a lounge chair and count the clouds or admire the azure blue sky.

+ Your home and (hopefully) work environment should be bright, light, and spacious.

+ Ideally sit or work near a window when you are indoors.

+ Try the 20-20-20 rule at work and at home when working on a screen, as recommended by the American Optometric Association, to reduce eye strain but also help with sleep issues: Look at something 20 feet away for at least 20 seconds every 20 minutes.

+ Eat at regular times because mealtimes are another zeitgeber (see page 65).

+ If you don't have access to natural light, then explore the use of artificial light boxes instead (see pages 69–70).

## EVENING

Minimize your exposure to bright or blue light, particularly in the few hours before you go to sleep:

+ Start by dimming your lights in the house about 3 hours before bedtime.

+ Do not look at bright screens ideally 2 to 3 hours before retiring, but if you can't, stop at least 45 minutes before.

+ If you have to use screens in the evening:
  - Use a blue light filter to change the color temperature of your display to a warmer tone, where possible.
  - Reduce the brightness to 50 percent or less.
  - Switch on the dark/night mode offered on certain apps or websites if available.

+ Aim to switch all main lights off about 1 to 2 hours before bedtime.

+ Use dimmed amber or red as bedside night-lights. Candlelight works, too, but make sure to blow out the candles before falling asleep.

+ Explore the Sleep Tech section on pages 177–187 for more guidance on smart lighting and blue light blocking solutions, including blue light filter apps, blue light-free light bulbs, and light-simulator alarm clocks.

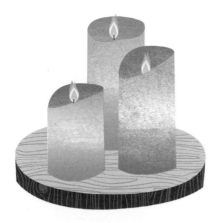

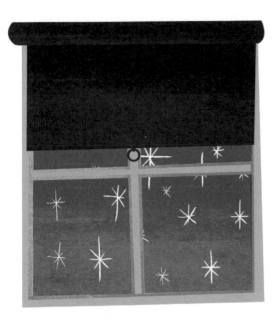

Note: *Night-shift workers will need to adapt their light regime to support their work pattern, using lighting to keep them alert.*

## OVERNIGHT

+ Keep your bedroom completely dark overnight by using blackout curtains or blinds.
+ As an alternative, use a comfortable eye mask but don't rely on airplane freebies—invest in a quality one that truly blocks out the light. It should be light and comfortably fit on your face.
+ Safely cover or hide any indicator lights, charger lights, or alarm clock displays.
+ Consider using a dawn simulator (also known as a wake-up light) to facilitate your awakening the next day.

## ABOUT LIGHT THERAPY

As explained on page 65, light is a powerful tool to reset the timing of the body clock to a healthy sleep–wake cycle. Light therapy is used effectively by scientists and doctors as a therapeutic instrument to treat seasonal affective disorders (SAD), depression, and to support night-shift work. Although more research is needed, light therapy has been shown to have a positive impact on sleep, more specifically to treat circadian rhythm disorders and temporary circadian disturbances. It can help us get more deep sleep, shift our wake-up time if needed, and improve our mood and performance during the day.

### WHITE OR BLUE LIGHT THERAPY

Medical SAD light boxes or lamps emit artificial white or blue light at an intensity of anywhere between 2,500 lux

CAUTION: *Light therapy can cause side effects for people with certain mental and eye health conditions.*

and 10,000 lux (units of illumination), which compares to 100,000–120,000 lux on a sunny day.

+ Light therapy should always be carried out under the supervision of a doctor.
+ Each light therapy session should last between 20 to 40 minutes.
+ It usually takes about 1 to 2 weeks for the treatment to take effect.
+ The timing and closeness to the source of light depends on the condition treated and should be prescribed by a medical professional.
+ Light usage guidelines for circadian rhythm disorders (DSPS, ASPS) and circadian rhythm disturbances (jet lag):
  - Use in the morning immediately after waking up to treat the Delayed Sleep Phase Syndrome (DSPS), which is falling asleep and waking up much later than acceptable, desired, or conventional.
  - Use in the evening before your usual bedtime to treat the Advanced Sleep Phase Syndrome (ASPS), which is falling asleep and waking up much earlier than acceptable, desired, or conventional.
  - Use upon awakening to minimize jet lag when traveling eastbound by bringing forward your wake-up time.
  - Use in the evening to minimize jet lag when traveling westbound by delaying sleep onset.
+ If a rack of lights is not convenient for you, opt for a desk lamp instead.
+ Shift workers can support their night shift by using such light in the evening to delay sleepiness. In this study looking at how to adapt the circadian rhythm of night-shift workers, the authors recommend the "combination of intermittent bright light during the night shift, sunglasses (as dark as possible) during the commute home, and a regular, early daytime sleep period in the dark."[4]

## OTHER LIGHT-THERAPY PRODUCTS

There are other products that release lighting that imitates natural light cycles, such as "sunrise" alarm clocks, wake-up light alarm clocks, and SAD alarm clocks. Their lighting will gradually increase from about 30 minutes before your desired wake-up time, which should make waking up easier and help make you feel more alert in the morning, avoiding a brutal alarm ringtone jolting you out of sleep. Some devices can also be programmed to decrease lighting gradually in the evening.

## RED LIGHT THERAPY

This is a debated therapeutic technique that uses red low-level wavelengths of light originally used for muscle recovery, wounds healing, injury recovery, and to treat skin issues by stimulating the regeneration of the skin. Studies have shown that it can also help improve sleep, as it as a warmer color temperature more likely to support melatonin production.[5]

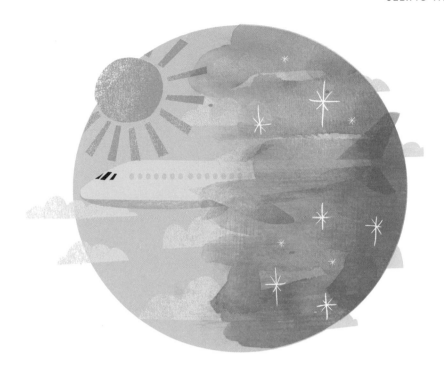

## MANAGING OCCASIONAL DISTURBANCES TO YOUR CIRCADIAN RHYTHM

When we travel in time, we expose ourselves to artificially created disturbances to our circadian rhythm. This is hardly science fiction or imaginary: when we change time zones, traveling long distances in a proportionately very short amount of time, our master clock is impacted and needs to adjust to the new day/dark-light cycle. This might also be true (although to a much lesser degree) when we save or gain 1 hour for daylight savings in the spring and fall.

### MANAGING JET LAG

We are all familiar with the dreadful feeling of jet lag when traveling to a different time zone, traveling into the future or back in time, when suddenly the days have become longer or shorter. We feel so drowsy and sleepy, sometimes nauseous, our stomach growls at odd hours, we are unable to think clearly or concentrate—it feels like just another day in the life of an insomniac.

This is the result of challenging our circadian rhythm to adjust to a new dark-light cycle before our body and brain are ready to do so. Our sleep and wake hormones are released at the usual time, while our sleep pressure also builds up as per our previous time zone.

Although it takes only a few days to adjust our rhythm, it takes 1 to 2 weeks for our wake-up hormone cortisol and our body temperature regulation to adjust. Light is our best ally to adapt and reset our body clock.

Here are some helpful tips to adjust to a new time zone:

+ Prepare gradually a few days before your departure: Delay sleep time if heading west, or go to bed earlier if traveling east.
  - If traveling east: Avoid bright evening lighting, go to bed early, set your alarm clock early, get up immediately, and head out for an outdoor workout. If you have access to a light box, use it in the morning to help you wake up.
  - If traveling west, keep bright lights or a light box on in the evening and go to bed later to prepare for staying awake later. If you land at night, then wake up at a normal time the next day, go outdoors immediately, or use a light box to reset.
+ Make sure you get plenty of rest before traveling—this will help you get over the jet lag faster on arrival.
+ Set all of your clocks and alarms to your new local time as soon as you board the plane.
+ Eat light meals, hydrate sufficiently, and avoid alcohol while traveling.
+ Upon arrival, follow the sunlight in your new location, staying awake until it gets dark, then sleep at least 4 to 5 hours during the local night.

+ Resist the temptation to take a long nap during the day, but if you have to, limit it to 30 minutes.
+ Avoid going to bed or waking up late.
+ Use a light box or bright lights if you struggle waking up at local time.
+ Eat your meals at the new local time.
+ Get as much sunlight as possible by spending time outdoors.
+ You may try taking melatonin supplements before bedtime to facilitate sleep onset. Results can vary depending on the individual.
+ Minimize all stimulants (caffeine, alcohol, cigarettes), especially in the evenings.
+ Use eye masks and earplugs to minimize sleep disruptions.

## DST—DAYLIGHT SAVING

Daylight saving was institutionalized so we can benefit from more daylight and save energy by shifting the time clock forward by an hour in spring and backwards an hour in the fall. Some argue, however, that this is causing unnecessary jet lag, increasing the risk to our health. If DST does affect you in this way and you are concerned about it, follow the jet-lag management tips for about a week to avoid any disturbances to your circadian rhythm.

+ Remember, it is easier to go to bed later than to wake up earlier, so it's always easier to travel westbound than eastbound! If it is a short trip then it is perhaps pointless to adjust to your new time zone, as you'd have to readjust again, so it might be best to keep your current timings and take short naps to manage daytime sleepiness.

+ Traveling at the crack of dawn? These tips also apply if you have to get up in the middle of the night to catch an early morning flight. Just practice by shifting your sleep earlier a few days before departing. Move your bedtime and wake up time half an hour earlier. Then move the times up by a further half hour the next day, and a further half hour the day after that.

+ On the plane or train:
  - Choose a good comfortable seat (leg room, reclining seat, window to lean your head on, away from possible disturbances).
  - Experiment with sleep accessories such as neck pillows, eye masks, and ear plugs.
  - Explore on-flight audio entertainment programs offering relaxing sounds, white noise, or playlists for sleep—and use noise-canceling headphones.

## ABOUT SOCIAL JET LAG

Do you go to bed or wake up later on weekends to catch up on sleep lost during the week? If so, you are experiencing "social jet lag," a term coined by chronobiologist Till Roenneberg to describe the way we schedule our sleep differently throughout the week, as opposed to following our natural circadian rhythm.[6] It might be by choice (going to a party or watching TV later than usual), or by necessity (working from home late). This results in an irregular sleep schedule with significant differences between work/school days and free days. This leads to accumulating a sleep debt which we believe can be recuperated over the weekend, but unfortunately this doesn't work if there is a long-term discrepancy between our social and biological needs. Doing so creates jet lag with consequences for your health and well-being. So, if you struggle with sleep, protect your circadian rhythm by observing the same wake up and bedtime every day of the week, even weekends, with rare exceptions.

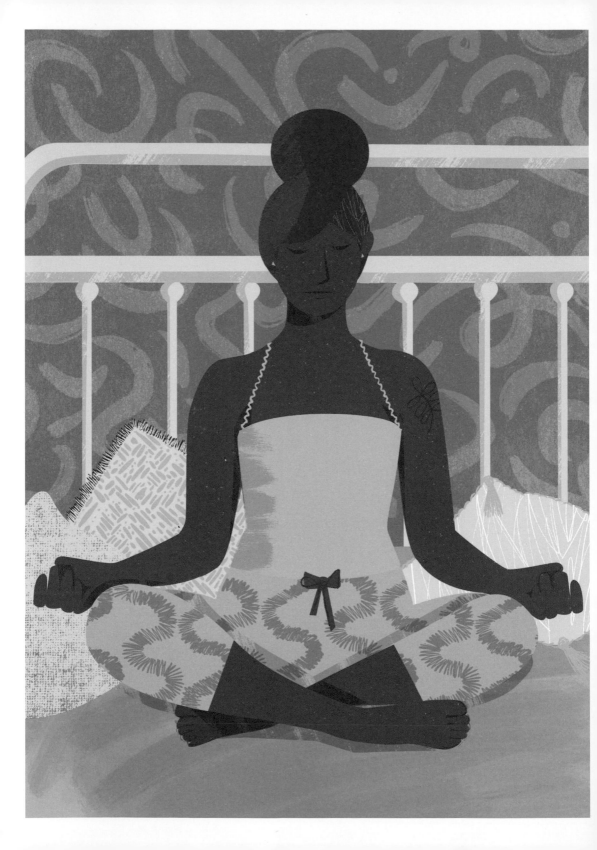

# BEDITATION

The term "beditation" originally meant to start your day with "a moment of morning mindlessness"[1] instead of waking up feeling agitated and worried. It has evolved to become a bedtime practice as well and is adopted widely by well-being practitioners and yoga instructors. The objective is to practice body, mind, and brain relaxation techniques in bed, right before you fall asleep, or as you gently wake up. Dreamy, isn't it? The techniques enable you to switch on the parasympathetic nervous system (see page 22) and manage obsessive thoughts, so you can fall asleep and manage overnight awakenings more easily.

## YOGA NIDRA

Yoga nidra, a restorative and deeply relaxing yoga practice, is a guided meditation that you can listen to on an app or other recording, while lying down completely relaxed. There are several restful yoga nidra poses, which you can practice in bed for 5 to 15 minutes.

"Shavasana" is the easiest yoga nidra pose and is easy to integrate into your nighttime routine:

Lie flat on your back, arms stretched out by your sides, palms faceup toward the ceiling, legs slightly apart, your body completely relaxed. Close your eyes and meditate or breathe deeply while slowly scanning and focusing on each part of your body to connect with the sensations there, such as tingling, numbness, or perhaps a feeling of warmth or coolness. Here are a few variations of the shavasana pose, all of which are simple to practice on a bed:

+ Elevate your legs with a pillow or place your feet against a wall at a 45-degree angle.
+ Bend your legs and let your knees fall outward with the soles of your feet touching.
+ Place a pillow underneath your upper back to open up the chest and abdomen.
+ Lie facedown with a comfortable support underneath your belly, ankles, or forehead, as needed.

---

CAUTION: If you have chronic insomnia (see page 36), avoid practicing these techniques in bed or in the bedroom. By keeping the bedroom strictly for sleep and intimacy, a stronger subconscious association will be created between sleep and bed. An exception might be the PMR technique (see pages 78–79) and breathing techniques while lying in bed, which should help you fall asleep more easily.

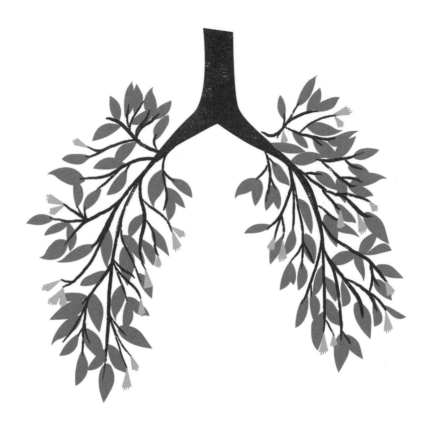

# BREATHWORK

Using breathing techniques is an excellent way to fall asleep. Controlled breathing acts as a natural off switch, calming the autonomic nervous system by stimulating the vagus nerve, which runs from your gut to your brain—this helps to activate the parasympathetic nervous system (see page 22).

Breathing in through the nose, slowly and deeply into the abdominal (belly) area, and breathing out even more slowly through the throat and mouth in particular, sends relaxation signals to the brain, helping to relieve physical, mental, and emotional tension, as well as slowing your heart rate. Conversely, rapid and shallow breathing sends stress signals to the brain. When you inhale, your heart rate naturally increases, and if you briefly hold your breath or exhale very slowly, your heart rate slows down—a normal physiological event that is linked to a state of relaxation. By breathing deeply before bedtime you imitate the slowing down breathing patterns that occur when you fall asleep. Do each breathwork technique for 5 to 10 minutes, depending on how quickly you feel relaxed and fall asleep.

## DOUBLE EXHALING

1. Breathe in deeply, breathe out twice as long.
2. Repeat until you feel deeply relaxed.

## 4–7–8 BREATHING

This breathing pattern technique, developed by Dr. Andrew Weil, is based on an ancient yogic technique called "pranayama."

1. Place your tongue against your palate, right behind your upper teeth.
2. Inhale deeply through your nose for 4 seconds.
3. Hold your breath for 7 seconds.
4. Exhale with a guttural sound such as "wooosh" or "aaah" quite audibly through your throat and mouth for 8 seconds.
5. Repeat this exercise until you fall asleep.

## ALTERNATE NOSTRIL BREATHING

Known as "nadi shodhana pranayama," this helps lower the heart rate and reduce stress. It is said to synchronize the two sides of the brain and purify the energy channels of the body. It is quite normal to have one side or the other congested or blocked, but do practice anyway until your blocked channel opens up naturally.

1. Exhale fully, then close the right nostril with your right thumb.
2. Inhale through your left nostril, then close the left nostril with your ring finger. Hold your breath very briefly.
3. Open your right nostril and exhale through it, while the left one is closed.
4. Inhale through the right nostril, then close it with your right thumb.
5. Release your ring finger and exhale through the left nostril. This is one cycle.
6. Continue this left-right rotation for 5 minutes, finishing by exhaling through your left nostril.
7. Start with 4 counts when breathing in and out and when holding your breath. Increase to 10 slow counts when you feel more experienced. Do not push yourself to hold your breath for longer if it creates anxiety or panic.

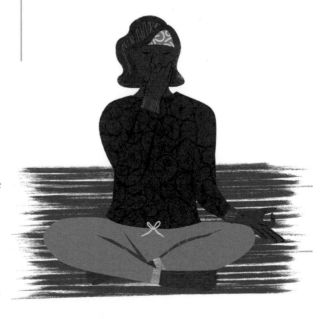

# MINDFULNESS OR MEDITATION TECHNIQUES

These practices usually require sitting down on the floor or on a chair, while staying alert. When used as beditation techniques, there are no restrictive rules—you will be sitting or lying down in bed and allowing yourself to gently drift off to sleep.

Mindfulness consists of clearing your thoughts while focusing your mind on the present moment and on current surroundings with kindness and acceptance. To find out more about Mindfulness, see the Taming Your Mind section on pages 87–95.

Meditation brings mental clarity in different ways: through visualization, by paying attention to the breath or the sensations in your body, by clearing all thoughts from the mind or observing them with no judgment or expectations. Some claim that a regular meditation or mindfulness practice results in needing less sleep. Others claim it increases alertness, so if you find the latter to be the case as you are trying to sleep, try a different beditation technique.

# PROGRESSIVE MUSCLE RELAXATION (PMR) TECHNIQUE

The principle of this highly effective relaxation technique is to contract then release each muscle group in turn, from head to toe, combined with focusing on your breathing. Tense each muscle group as vigorously as possible, then completely release the tension while breathing out simultaneously until you feel each body part sink into the bed. Keep the focus on contracting, releasing, and breathing, and be gentle with any painful areas of your body. Contract each muscle for 5–10 counts, hold for 5–10 counts, then release for 5–10 counts, allowing the tension to fall away time after time in the following muscle group order:

1. Lie in bed, hands by your sides, feet hip-distance apart.
2. Tighten the muscles in your forehead (frown), hold, then abruptly relax and breathe out.
3. Now close your eyes and squeeze your eyelids firmly, hold, then release them as if they are slightly floating upward, then breathe out.
4. Clench your mouth and jaw for a moment, hold, then let them go very soft and breathe out.
5. Smile widely, stretching your mouth and cheeks, hold, then let go.
6. Tilt your head backward and scrunch the back of your neck as tight as possible, hold, then release, feeling

the tension melt away.

7. Raise your shoulders as high as possible toward your ears, hold, then release and breathe, feeling them sink into the mattress.

8. Clench your fists and tense both arms, hold, then relax letting them go completely limp, and breathe out.

9. Inhale deeply into your lungs at maximum capacity, hold your breath, then slowly exhale all the tension out of your chest.

10. Contract and suck in your stomach muscles as vigorously as possible, hold, then relax and breathe out.

11. Gently raise and arch the small of your back off your bed, hold, then release and breathe out.

12. Tense your buttocks, hold, then let go abruptly and breathe out, imagining sinking into the mattress.

13. Tense both legs pointing your toes forward, hold, then suddenly relax and breathe out and feel the weight of your legs sink into the mattress.

With your body completely relaxed from head to toe, inhale into your belly, deeply and slowly, then breathe out as deeply as you can, with your stomach sinking toward your spine. If it helps, place your hand on your stomach during this exercise, letting your body sink into the bed after each exhale, each time feeling a little heavier and more relaxed. Repeat the deep breathing until you fall asleep. If you don't make it to step 13 before you fall asleep, that's good!

## THE BODY-SCAN MEDITATION

A simple and effective way to achieve ultimate relaxation in bed is to mentally scan your body from head to toe, slowly and progressively. The principle is similar to PMR (see above), but without the muscle contraction. The technique is to imagine a circle of light surrounding and scanning your whole body and as it travels slowly up and down, notice any areas of tension. Stay with those areas until they relax, one by one. Follow the same order from head to toe as for PMR. You are likely to experience physical sensations such as tingling, aching, tickling, pulsating, vibrating, pressure, pain, cold or heat, and so on. This is perfectly normal as this technique heightens and isolates physical sensations, but these should come and go as you move through the surface and depth of the body.

# MUDRAS

In yoga practice, "mudras" are hand gestures that activate the energetic circuits and channels within our body and are believed to facilitate energy flow while stimulating our emotions and bodily responses. Positioning the fingers in different ways connects the hands to specific areas of the brain, stimulating reflexes, internal glands, and physiological functions. By doing each mudra in conjunction with focusing on the breath increases the energy flow in the body, impacting on the sensory organs, tendons, glands, and veins. Practicing mudras by itself or in conjunction with another relaxation or beditation technique, wherever practical, could help your daily energy flow and help regulate your brain and biological functions toward better sleep. Practice daily for 5-15 minutes. Here are three for you to try:

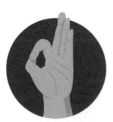

### GYAN MUDRA:
*Mudra of Knowledge*

Press the tips of the thumb and index finger together keeping the other three fingers straight. This activates the pituitary and endocrine glands. You can practice while in bed and throughout the day.

BENEFITS: *Helps to ease insomnia, sharpens the brain, enhances memory and concentration, reduces anxiety.*

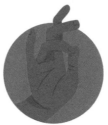

### SURYA MUDRA:
*Mudra of the Sun*

With your palm face up, bend your ring finger and press it down with your thumb. This connects with the thyroid gland.

BENEFITS: *Helps to reduce anxiety, weight, and cholesterol, and improves all digestive functions.*

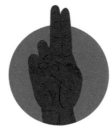

### PRANA MUDRA:
*Mudra of Life*

Bend the ring finger and the little finger and press them with the tip of your thumb, keeping the remaining two fingers straight. This revitalizes energy into the body and stimulates internal organs. This one can be practiced daily at any time and for any duration.

BENEFITS: *Helps to improve immunity, relieve fatigue, reduce vitamin deficiency.*

# VISUALIZATION

Visualization is an enjoyable technique to take you away from the obsessive, stressful, and random thoughts that can get in the way of your sleep. It is particularly effective after completing PMR (see pages 78–79) or body scanning (see page 79). You simply picture an imaginary, pleasing place, and fully engage your five senses—sight, smell, touch, hearing, taste—noticing every detail of your surroundings and watching yourself evolve within them. It helps to decide in advance what you are going to visualize, so you don't have to overthink think this as you are trying to sleep. Choose whichever settings or scenes seem most soothing to you. Visualization can be done before sleep or if you wake during the night. As well as creating your own, you can try listening to guided visualizations on an app or download a recording (see page 183).

## PICTURING SLEEP

To demonstrate the power of imagery in relation to sleep, a study[2] was conducted in 2002 exposing a group of insomniacs to a stressor. They were instructed to think about giving a speech in either images or verbal thoughts (words). The findings were that in the longer term, the image group estimated that they fell asleep more quickly and, the following morning, reported less anxiety and more comfort about giving the speech compared with the verbal group.

In his book *Relax and Win: Championship Performance In Whatever You Do*, Bud Winter shares visualization techniques that are apparently employed by the US military, and that will help you to relax and fall asleep within 2 minutes. Following muscular relaxation, you visualize lying in a canoe with the clear blue sky above your head or lying in a velvet black hammock in a pitch-dark room.

# MIND FOCUS

We tend to feel increasingly anxious in the evening as night falls. It is most likely evolutionary: since we are not nocturnal beings and our vision is naturally very low at night, we have an innate alert system to watch out for predators as darkness comes on. Ancestral predators are now replaced by stressful thoughts about the pressures of modern life. These thoughts tend to be more prevalent in the evening when everything slows down. They are loud, can become obsessive, and prevent us from sleeping. See the section called Taming the Mind (see pages 87-95) for techniques to help you cope, but also try these easy beditation techniques to focus your mind:

## THE EYES-WIDE-OPEN TECHNIQUE

This technique is based on reverse psychology, also called paradoxical intention. A study[3] requiring insomniacs to force themselves to stay awake showed a significant reduction in sleep effort and sleep performance anxiety. The trick is to make a conscious effort to keep your eyes open and stay awake for as long as possible, while lying in your bed in the dark. Ideally look up at the ceiling and make every effort not to close your eyes, except for blinking, even if this means doing so for hours. This method can help you fall asleep faster than you can imagine and quieten the mind, even though it makes you more sensitive to external stimuli. By focusing your attention on keeping the eyes open and being determined not to sleep, the technique heightens the urge to sleep. It is quite a sensory experience, and you will get better at it with time and practice, even if you consciously know and understand why it works.

## " THE"

Another way to distract the mind without stimulating the brain is to repeat a neutral word such as "the." This type of word doesn't have any connotation or imagery attached to it when used on its own, yet it gives a sense of focus. It can be repeated over and over mentally, or out loud (if that is an option).

---

CAUTION: Do not take any stimulants such as coffee or alcohol to try the eyes-wide-open technique. Discontinue if it does not work for you after being awake for hours.

# POSITION YOUR BODY FOR BETTER SLEEP

As part of beditation, it is worth looking at our sleep positions. As we lie down, we soon need to adopt a comfortable position to be able to sleep. We might toss and turn until we find it, or we might always sleep in the same position out of habit. The reality is that no matter how we fall asleep, we will naturally shift our positions many times during the night. Certain positions can worsen some medical issues such as sleep apnea (see page 37), and chronic back or shoulder pain, which will prompt even more changes in sleep positions throughout the night. Most of us switch from lying on our backs to lying on either side during non-REM phases of sleep when we are not in a state of sleep paralysis.

Here are a few positions for optimal comfort, but of course only you will know what is best for you based on how refreshed and pain-free you feel the next day. It is useful to remember that it is best to position yourself with your spine in a natural alignment. Do not force a position upon yourself if it doesn't suit you or creates pain or discomfort.

## SUPINE POSITION

If you sleep flat on your back, place a pillow underneath your knees to reduce pressure and relieve musculoskeletal pain. Make sure it is not higher than the height of two fists on top of each other. In addition, position your head on a curved ergonomic pillow (see page 60), with the thicker part underneath the bottom of your neck. The pillows will help to keep the spine relatively neutral and the lower back slightly curved while alleviating pressure on the joints. The drawback of this position is that it can worsen snoring and obstructive sleep apnea.

## SIDE POSITION

If you are a side sleeper, consider placing a pillow (not too thick) between your knees, folded slightly upward to help with spine alignment and neutral pelvic position. This position can help ease breathing and can be beneficial to those with lower back pain and to pregnant women, as it reduces pressure on the bladder. However, it can put pressure on certain organs depending on which side you sleep, and can create shoulder, lower back, and hip pain.

## STOMACH POSITION

If you must sleep on your stomach because it feels good to you, consider making these adjustments to help reduce lower back and neck pain and facilitate breathing:

+ Place a pillow underneath your chest or head.
+ Place another pillow under your lower abdomen and upper pelvic area.
+ Make sure both pillows are no thicker than 3 inches, as comfortable to you.

If it is still uncomfortable, remove the pillow from underneath your chest/head, or use an even thinner one. Be aware that this position might impact your blood circulation and breathing.

## THE CANAL FOR SHOULDER PAIN

In this position, using a combination of pillows provides support for the neck and head while creating an open "canal" space where the shoulder and arm can be placed without feeling as much pressure. Lying on your side, stack a couple of comfortable pillows under your head, and one underneath your torso, leaving a space between the two.

## SLEEPING UPRIGHT

Certain specialized beds and mattresses can be adjusted in terms of feet and head elevation at the touch of a remote control. Another more affordable way is to use a large wedge pillow. Raising the upper body should most likely reduce snoring and sleep apnea. This position should also help with lumber pain, but it will be difficult to shift to any other position during the night.

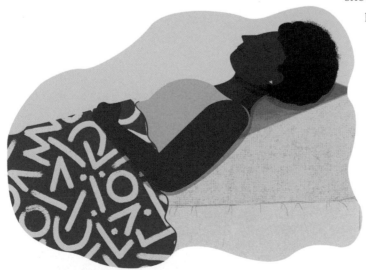

# WHY SEX CAN BE GOOD FOR SLEEP

Engaging in sexual activity generates the feel-good hormone oxytocin, which is essential for our well-being. Sex is a form of exercise, with intense muscular contraction and release and heavy breathing, so not dissimilar to the PMR technique (see pages 78–79)—in a sense, it is a natural form of beditation! There is little doubt that the vagus nerve that helps us sleep (see page 22) is also stimulated during sex.

There is a close relationship between sleeping and sex and it's not just that both seem to take place generally in a bed or that "sleeping with someone" means having sex with them. Sex hormones are released at their highest levels during REM sleep. REM stages happen several times during the night and get longer in duration in the second half of the night. If you cut your night's sleep short, this eats into

REM sleep, which would be, among other things, detrimental to the production of sex hormones.

Good sleep is proven to help increase the libido and desire for sex, and there is a strong connection between sleep and orgasms. While men have "wet" dreams and erections, women experience clitoral engorgement and nocturnal orgasms during REM sleep stages. Studies have shown that both genders experienced potentially more intense orgasms during sleep than awake, possibly because there are fewer psychological and emotional barriers when sleeping.

Generally speaking, having sex and orgasms seems to give us quality sleep right after the effort of climaxing, and often for the rest of the night as well.

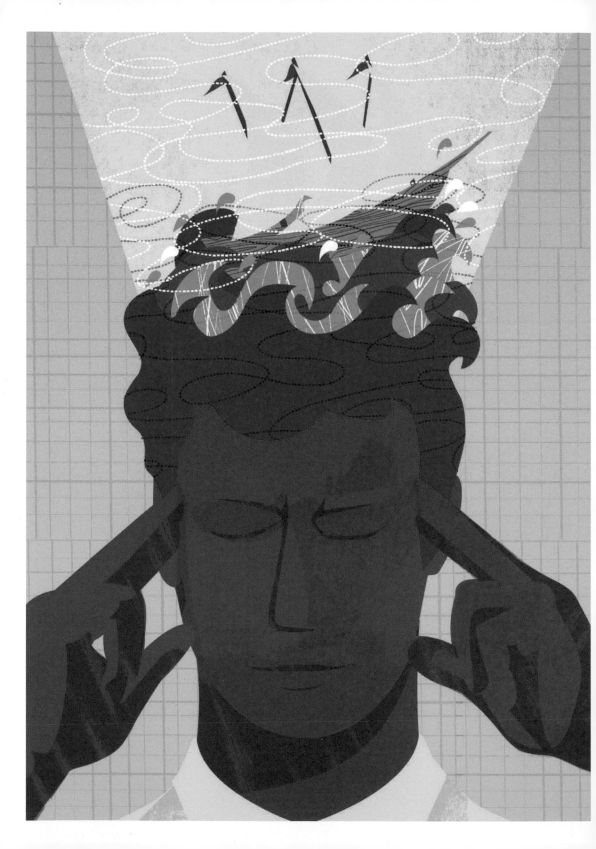

# TAMING THE MIND

Sleep is orchestrated by the brain and works wonders overnight for both brain and body, yet it is perhaps our mind that has the greatest influence over our sleep. Our mind grants us the gift of awareness, consciousness, thoughts, and feelings, yet it wants to run wild from time to time and is often the main cause of sleep disruption. Sleep deprivation also impacts on our mental health and psychological well-being; in particular, individuals with depression or anxiety are more likely to suffer from insomnia. In this section, we explore psychological and behavioral therapies, techniques, and practices designed to tame the mind for a good night's sleep.

## OUR THINKING MIND

Every day we have between 50,000–90,000 thoughts and we might feel several of the 27 distinct categories of emotions as identified by scientists at the University of California, Berkeley. No wonder it can sometimes get difficult to manage our thoughts, and more specifically, negative thoughts.

In fact, a study showed that having repetitive negative thoughts is associated with shorter sleep duration and delayed sleep timing.[1] Another study concluded that "high intention to fall asleep worsened sleep quality, especially in terms of sleep fragmentation, in good sleepers,"[2] which means the more effort we put into thinking about getting good sleep, the less likely it is to happen.

Stress, worries, and anxiety are major sleep disrupters as well. When we are stressed or anxious, our body releases high levels of the stress hormone cortisol throughout the day and the night causing us to have shorter and restless sleep.

This interferes with our circadian rhythm as it fails to make us feel relaxed or active at the appropriate time of the sleep-wake cycle.

In the United States, 77 percent of people regularly experience physical symptoms caused by stress, according to the American Institute of Stress, which means that most of us are likely to experience stress-related sleep issues. A Stress in America™ survey showed that 45 percent of Americans feel even more stressed if they do not get enough sleep.[3]

Let's review some of the mind management techniques that can help us achieve better sleep.

# BEHAVIORAL TECHNIQUES FOR SLEEP

Behavioral therapy aims to identify and eliminate unhealthy or unhelpful behaviors that create problems in our lives. The principles behind this therapeutic approach are that behaviors are learned and acquired from our circumstances, our upbringing, our environment, and the events that happen in our lives. But behaviors can be changed with concrete actions, undoing the bad ones and learning new ones, with focus and commitment. In the context of sleep therapy, it is both about the way we do things and the way we think about situations.

## COGNITIVE BEHAVIORAL THERAPY FOR INSOMNIA (CBTI)

CBTi is the most proven and established method of curing insomnia. It is a combination of lifestyle adjustments, behavioral changes, mind-management techniques, and tailored sleep scheduling. It is inspired by, but different from, CBT, specifically addressing a wide range of sleep issues and disorders.

The CBTi technique is taught in five or more sessions, supervised by a sleep consultant. It consists of:

+ Understanding the sleep–wake process.
+ Filling out a sleep diary to monitor the average time spent sleeping and calculate sleep efficiency based on your time in bed versus hours actually spent sleeping.
+ Adopting stricter sleep hygiene (nutrition, avoiding stimulants, limited exposure to blue light, exercise, sleep-promoting environment, and habits).
+ Following these key CBTi principles:
  - Aim to wake up and get up at the same time every day, even at weekends.
  - Avoid napping.
  - Follow the 15-minute rule. Rather than tossing and turning indefinitely, leave the bedroom if you are still awake in bed after 15 minutes, and come back when you feel sleepy. Repeat as needed.
  - Implement stimulus control: This practical technique is designed to create an exclusive subconscious connection between sleep and the bed, banning all activities from the bedroom other than sleep and sexual activity.
  - Move all waking activities outside the bedroom, including meditating, reading, watching TV, talking on the phone, listening to music, texting or surfing the web, eating, exercising, working, and the list goes on.
  - Implement sleep scheduling: Restricting sleep duration to improve the quality of sleep, before gradually increasing its duration. This methodology is complex and definitely requires professional supervision.
+ Practice relaxation and the thought-management techniques below to help ease insomnia.
+ Observe a wind-down routine designed to create a buffer between your active day and sleep, during which you evaluate your day objectively and identify the next day's projects.

# MANAGING STRESSFUL THOUGHTS

Thoughts can make us feel pressured, stressed, fearful, anxious, and give us a sense of urgency or a loss of control. Therefore it is important to process difficult thoughts and emotions ahead of bedtime so we can go to sleep with a quiet mind. Here are some helpful techniques to do so. Note that they are most effective when done in writing on paper:

+ Keep a personal journal with your thoughts, reflections, and worries, and write in it a few hours before sleep, recognizing what went badly and acknowledging any negative thoughts, alongside what went well and positive thoughts.
+ Use the below "evaluation balance sheet" method and look at each situation through the following filter:
  - What is the situation?
  - How do I feel about it?
  - Why is this happening?
  - Evidence that confirms my belief
  - Alternative evidence that contradicts my belief
  - How do I feel about this after evaluation?
+ Practice gratitude and appreciation for the good things in our lives.
+ Do not worry about sleep as it will only make it worse, especially while you are lying in bed. Do not try to force sleep. Change the narrative by believing that sleep will come if you relinquish control and let it happen.
+ Set aside some time for conscious worrying long before bedtime, outside the bedroom for 5 to 15 minutes every day, or as needed. List all of your worries on paper.
+ Then apply the "control technique": establish what you have direct control over, what others control but you can influence, and areas that concern you but over which you have no control— such as past and future events or wider problems. Once you have identified your position, make an action plan to tackle the issues, keeping in mind how much control you have over the situation.
+ Prepare the following day or week ahead, outlining your priorities, projects, tasks and actions to move things forward and resolve difficult situations.

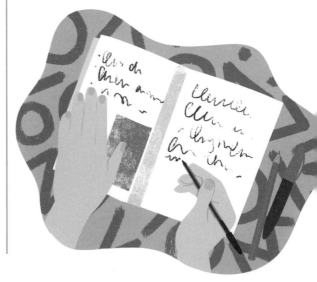

# MANAGING OBSESSIVE THOUGHTS

If during the night you have an obsessive thought, or FOMO (fear of missing out), try these simple techniques:

+ Use a "thought algorithm," processing each thought through the following questions:
  - Is this thought useful (yes/no)?
  - Can I do something about it now? (yes/no)?
  - Can I do it as well or better tomorrow or another day? If yes, schedule a day and time to do it. If no, get out of bed and do it right away.
  *Note: It is best to write in your journal as you work through this technique to lighten your brain.*

+ Try one of these thought-clearing techniques:
  - The eyes-wide-open technique while lying down in the dark (see page 82).
  - Saying "the" as a thought-stopping technique (see page 82).
  - The "stepping out of the thought" technique, based on mindfulness and acceptance and commitment therapy (ACT— see page 95), to create perspective and distance from the thought by saying "I notice I am having the thought that (then state your negative thought)."

# MIND-CONTROL PRACTICES

The following techniques are great for clarity and focus, to make us feel relaxed, and to help shut down the noise and complexities of our lives for a moment. Make time for a daily practice, whether based on imagery, the breath, or sensations in the body. You can practice on your own, choose to be guided by an instructor, or use a recording if easier. Each of these techniques requires patience and training to optimize the results.

## VISUALIZATION

With the simple technique of visualization you use your mind to fully immerse yourself in an imaginary environment or scene, filled with detailed images and vivid sensations. You are likely to feel calm and experience well-being within minutes. Use your imagination or let yourself be guided by an instructor.

Once in a relaxed position, envision a world of your own in great descriptive detail, ideally engaging your five senses: touch, smell, taste, hearing, sight. This scene could be visualizing someone walking their dog on the beach from afar, yourself swinging on a hammock with a cold fruity drink in hand, or you and your partner walking hand in hand through a countryside field on a sunny day feeling a warm breeze over your arms, seeing wildflowers all around you.

The key is to choose your favorite imaginary scene in advance, so you can instantly transport yourself there without any effort as you try to fall asleep. Then take your time to explore and feel all the details of this vivid, relaxing, and comforting scene.

## MEDITATION

Meditation can be defined as the ability to clear your mind of all thoughts or to focus your attention on a single thing, avoiding rumination, intentional thinking, or reasoning. It is practiced as mind training, a relaxation technique, or as a spiritual practice. It requires self-awareness and the ability to connect to your inner self, to a life force, or to the universe. Although meditation requires you to stay alert, it slows down your brain waves so that you are in a deeply relaxed state which helps your brain get ready for sleep.

In fact, some meditation leaders say that meditators do not need as much sleep as non-meditators.

All meditation techniques have in common that, like sleep, they sharpen our brain, our memory, and make us feel deeply relaxed, less reactive to difficult emotions, and happier in life. In fact, when monitoring brain activity, scientists observed that the amygdala (the part of the brain responsible for emotions,

stress, and fight and flight) is less reactive to images with emotional content than after having meditated for 8 weeks.[4]

There are many different styles of meditation:

- Eyes closed, half open, or fully open looking at the horizon.
- Self practice or guided by an instructor.
- Silent or chanting mantras.
- With a natural or a forced breathing pattern.
- Sitting, walking, moving, or lying down.
- Focusing on either the breath or a mental image.
- As guided imagery meditation, which is similar to visualization.
- Scanning the sensations of the body or engaging the five senses.
- Spiritual practice or training for the mind.
- Clearing thoughts or observing your thoughts float away.

## MINDFULNESS

Mindfulness or mindful meditation consists of consciously observing yourself and your surroundings, staying in the present moment, focusing on the breath, and watching your thoughts and emotions without any judgment. You should notice small changes and events around you. Even if your mind wanders, traveling through the past and future, the key is to stay aware and fully present. This can be practiced quietly or while doing any activity, like walking, eating, traveling, doing chores.

Mindfulness helps to release tension and anxiety, and this simple and effective practice has become so popular that you can find many techniques explained in books, online, on apps, or even take classes.

## VIPASSANA

"Vipassana," an ancient Indian meditation technique, guides us to see things as they are, by observing ourselves, breathing naturally, and experiencing the law of impermanence, which means that nothing stays the same. The aim is to eradicate all suffering, addictions, mood disorders, stress, anguish, and psychosomatic ailments by accepting everything as it is. Vipassana meditation aims to liberate individuals toward full enlightenment by eliminating craving, aversion, and ignorance with regular and diligent practice. While its principles were developed by the Buddha, vipassana is non-denominational and not religious, therefore does not conflict with any faiths and it is for everyone, not only Buddhists.

# PSYCHO-EMOTIONAL HEALING THERAPIES

The following therapies tap into the mind-body connection and seem to give relief, a sense of well-being, and sometimes even profound healing to sleepless individuals.

## HYPNOSIS

This term comes from the Greek language *hypnos* meaning "sleep" and *-osis* meaning condition. It refers to an interaction where a hypnotist verbally influences someone's thoughts, perception, feelings, sensations, and behavior by getting them to focus on related images, concepts, and ideas. These therapeutic suggestions are made while the person is in a deeply relaxed state. Hypnosis is often combined with guided imagery, and sometimes with sounds or breathing exercises. Age regression is a common procedure, where the hypnotist guides the patient back in time to relive a past experience. Self-hypnosis is when the suggestions are self-created or learned through hypnotic instruction.

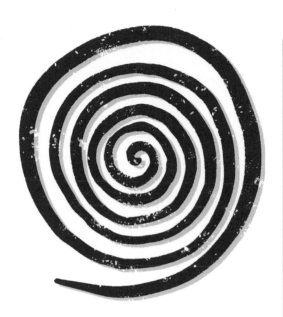

## NEURO-HYPNOTIC REPATTERNING (NHR®)

This is another technique designed to rewire the neural pathways and release the natural neuro-chemicals that make you feel good. The objective is to change default or negative thinking patterns and belief systems. The NHR® therapist uses a hypnotic process to facilitate the slowing down of the brain waves to a theta level, between the awake and light sleep states, incorporating breathwork, guided imagery, and soft music (or sounds). The voice-over script is filled with positive suggestions, thoughts, images, desires, and wishes, bringing back the patient feeling energized, positive, and relaxed.

## EMOTIONAL FREEDOM THERAPY (EFT)

Also called tapping, this technique is designed to remove emotional blocks and rewire our thinking patterns to clear unwanted thoughts, feelings, and beliefs. The most effective way to clear them and remove the blockages stored in our bodies is by gently tapping on specific points repetitively in a specific order, while acknowledging verbally what you are feeling and that you accept yourself unconditionally. Combined with deep breathing, this technique has the power to make you feel lighter and relieved.

## 5-4-3-2-1 COPING (GROUNDING) TECHNIQUE FOR ANXIETY

This is a technique using your five senses, one by one, noticing your surroundings to overcome anxiety. Noticing 5 things you can touch, 4 things you can see, 3 things you can hear, 2 things you can smell, 1 thing you can taste. The senses and numbers are interchangeable.

## AUTOGENIC THERAPY

Autogenic therapy is a self-help method learned over 8 to 10 weeks, providing deep physical and mental relaxation. It is effective at reducing stress, anxiety, tension, pain, and relieving insomnia. It combines exercises focusing on the sensations in different parts of the body, especially sensations of warmth and gravity, with visual imagery, verbal suggestions, and mind focus. This technique is similar to self-hypnosis and activates the parasympathetic nervous system, needed to fall asleep. It can be practiced anywhere and anytime, from a half a minute to half an hour.

## SOPHROLOGY

Sophrology is a technique blending Western and Eastern philosophies such as yoga, Buddhist meditation, and Japanese Zen, with techniques such as hypnosis, visualization, mindfulness, breathing exercises, gentle movements, tension-release, and awareness of different parts of your body. Sophrology therapists believe this method is very efficient to get more deep sleep.

# SPIRITUAL PRACTICES

For some of us, finding peace of mind means turning to a spiritual or religious practice for guidance and support. Prayers, spiritual meditation, and chanting, as well as spiritual or faith-based ceremonies, can have a powerful effect on emotional well-being, lift our spirits, and help us sleep. In particular, closing the day with such a practice is a way to reflect, show gratitude, and let go of worries and the difficult situations you might have faced during the day, even if it is just for a moment before sleep. Practiced alone or with your family members, it can be a soul-searching moment that gives a sense of protection, direction, and inner happiness as a way to wind down and prepare for peaceful slumber.

Some will invoke their god, the universe, mantras, spirits, or energetic forces. Some believe that the reason for poor sleep lies in past lives or being held back energetically by previous relationships and making them feel tormented. If this inspires you, you might want to explore "past life regression" in a therapeutic setting to recover memories and traumas of previous lives. This technique involves investigating someone while hypnotized, asking a series of questions to reveal identity and events of past lives.

Another one is "cord-cutting," a therapeutic ritual designed to break the energetic attachments we built with someone else, allowing us to move on and free ourselves from unhealthy or unproductive relationships, whether romantic or not.

# PSYCHOTHERAPEUTIC SUPPORT

Sometimes, our inability to sleep sufficiently is linked to deeply rooted psychological issues that need unearthing professionally. It could be trauma, bereavement, depression, anxiety, stress, fears, or phobias. In that case, look into getting guidance, support, or treatment from a professional coach, counselor, psychotherapist, psychologist, or a psychiatrist for more serious mental health conditions.

## TALK THERAPIES

Speech and words have the power to hurt or to heal. Actively and consciously sharing our struggles, concerns, or anxieties with a professional therapist goes a long way to alleviate the pain. You can speak confidentially and safely with someone professionally trained in a way that you couldn't with someone close. There are many types of talk therapies, perhaps the four most relevant to ease sleep issues are:

### PSYCHOTHERAPEUTIC COUNSELING

This is sharing your issues with a professional counselor to be able to come to terms with a difficult or troubling situation or understanding your patterns when it comes to your relationships with others.

### COGNITIVE BEHAVIORAL THERAPY (CBT)

This gives you the confidence to share your issues verbally, identify the behaviors that are possibly causing

you to be unhappy, and learn ways to change them; for example you may see a situation from an alternative perspective or adopt new strategies to deal with the situation at hand.

### TRAUMA THERAPY

This is a type of mental health treatment to overcome psychological trauma, which is caused by past events perceived as grave danger by our conscious and subconscious brain, putting us in constant alert mode. The most common form of trauma is post-traumatic stress disorder, or PTSD, an anxiety disorder with severe symptoms, such as flashbacks and insomnia. Treatment for this condition is complex, which is why therapists use a combination of techniques such as CBT, EFT (see page 93), and methods to challenge the belief system, or prolong exposure to the source of trauma. The patient safely faces the reality of the event without being a prisoner of it.

### ACCEPTANCE AND COMMITMENT THERAPY (ACT)

Most often combined with mindfulness, acceptance and commitment therapy supports you in facing your feelings and thoughts as opposed to avoiding or pushing back on them, even if they are difficult. The idea is to accept what you are not in control of and commit to behavioral changes to improve your life and become more resilient and psychologically adaptable.

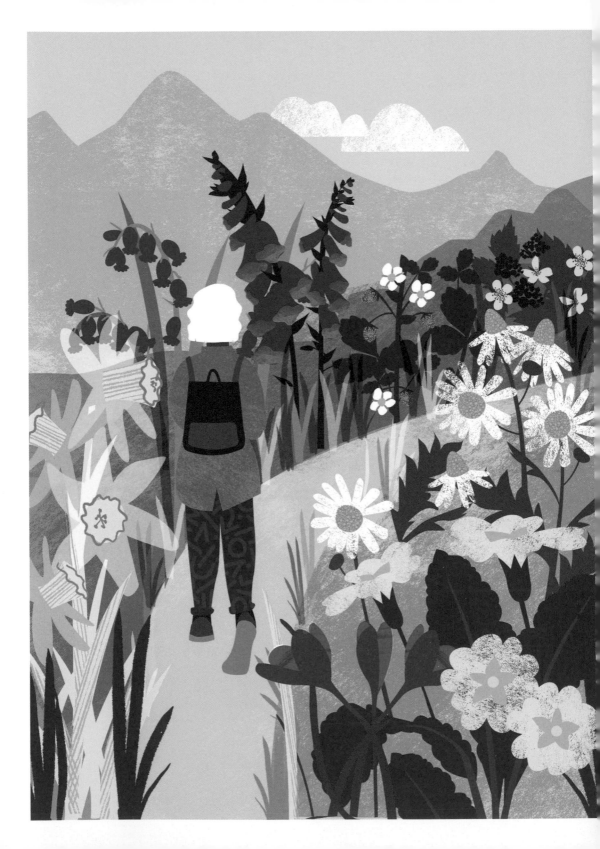

# GENTLE MOVEMENT

Leading a sedentary lifestyle is generally not good for well-being. Our mental and physical health very much depend on daytime activity, and so does our sleep. As diurnal beings, the more active we are in the day, especially outdoors, the more likely we are to achieve proper rest and recovery during the night. This is most likely evolutionary, as our ancestors were active during the day, hunting, gathering, and running away from danger. In this section you will find guidance on how to exercise for better sleep and channel your physical energy effectively, as well as how sleep supports your physical recovery and performance, whether at a gentle or athletic level.

## THE RIGHT EXERCISE FOR YOU

"Gentle movement" is about finding out what works for you. The answer is not always about pushing yourself too hard to achieve better sleep—more gentle forms of exercise can be just as effective. Choosing the optimal time of day and type(s) of exercise for you will play an instrumental role in the duration and quality of your sleep.

## EXERCISE TO SLEEP

Scientific studies generally support the theory that we are guaranteed to sleep soundly after a good workout, but some give conflicting results depending on age and particular circumstances, as well as the type and timing of exercise. Still, there is mounting evidence that regular exercise supports our physiological, hormonal, and metabolic processes as well as our mental health and our nervous system toward more and better sleep.

Exercising daily for 20 to 30 minutes (or at least 3 to 4 times a week) for 12 to 16 weeks, has been scientifically proven to improve sleep quality and duration for the majority of people. It is particularly effective when exercising outdoors, exposed to natural sunlight, especially between 10 am and 4 pm. Research shows that exposure to light combined with our body temperature cooling down after exercise, and the positive impact of exercise on our sympathetic nervous system (see page 22) and moods may be the perfect combination to make us sleep, especially in older adults.[1]

Exercise supports your health and sleep by eliminating toxins, releasing body tension, and maintaining a good weight (which is particularly helpful for sleep apnea in case of obesity). It also boosts energy while depleting cortisol levels, which means we don't go to sleep with high levels of the stress hormone in our system. Exercise releases endorphins, which can also relieve chronic pain and make us feel good, all of which are conducive to a good night's sleep.

## SLEEP TO EXERCISE

Conversely, sleep is essential to exercise. Experts believe that human growth hormone (HGH or GH) is released during stage N3 slow-wave sleep (see page 18), our deepest sleep. GH supports our body composition, cell repair, growth, recovery, and metabolism, and also boosts muscle growth, strength, and exercise performance. Being sleep deprived results in not feeling motivated to exercise or able to perform at your best physically. A lack of sleep also impacts on learning skills, strength, vigilance, concentration, and energy levels, all of which can lead to poor physical performance and a higher risk of injury. Today's athletes are prioritizing their sleep to ensure peak performance.

## TICKTOCK—WHAT TIME THEN?

You will need to experiment to figure out the best time of day to exercise for your own sleep duration and quality, but any time of day is better than not doing it at all. Here are some findings stemming from several scientific studies:

+ The timing of exercise can impact your circadian rhythms (body clock), by possibly shifting it.
+ Exercising earlier in the day may improve the quality of sleep.
+ Morning exercise seems to reduce the time it takes to fall asleep.
+ A cardio activity in the morning may result in more deep sleep.[2]
+ Strength training at any time of the day may improve sleep. Those who do so in the morning tend to fall asleep faster than those who work out later in the day, and those lifting weights in the evening are less likely to wake up frequently during the night and sleep better overall, in comparison with those who train early in the day.
+ Exercising in the afternoon or later may help reduce insomnia by lessening arousal (making you less stimulated/alert), anxiety, and depression.
+ Working out intensively too close to bedtime may overstimulate your nervous system, speed up your heart rate, and raise your blood pressure, leading to exacerbated wakefulness, alertness, an increased body temperature, and a boost in cortisol and adrenaline. This can make it difficult for some people to unwind and sleep through the night. Experiment with exercising vigorously in the evening, but not in the 2 hours before bedtime. It's important to allow a sufficient cool-down period for your body temperature to drop and return

to normal before you go to bed. A few tips for the wind-down: Do some gentle stretches, have a warm shower then cool the water temperature; open your windows to allow cool air into the bedroom.

# WHICH FORM OF EXERCISE SHOULD I CHOOSE?

Any activity is better than none, and the reality is that experts know little about how much and what forms of exercise promote sleep the most, especially for chronic insomniacs. So commit to the exercise of your choice, whether active or gentle, and discover for yourself how it impacts your sleep. Here is some guidance:

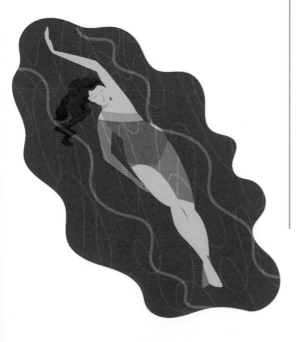

+ Regular moderate aerobic exercise has been proven to improve sleep. That is any activity that increases your heart rate, such as paced walking, running, cycling, rowing, or swimming.
+ Strength training such as lifting weights is thought to help you get better sleep because muscle growth and deep sleep are interdependent. Sleep itself promotes tissue repair, growth, healing, and recovery.
+ Yoga blends many benefits: low-impact physical exercise, strength and flexibility training, breath and relaxation, mental focus and meditative flow, all of which reduce stress, tension, and anxiety, while channeling our internal energy and our ability to feel good, and engaging our parasympathetic nervous system (see page 22).
+ Yoga nidra (or yogic sleep), in particular, is a form of meditation facilitating relaxation, rest, and recovery with comfortable poses and minimal effort, other than being guided into a full body scan and awareness of the breath (see page 75).
+ Pre-bedtime stretches are also a great way to relax and prepare for slumber. Whether neck side pulls, shoulder rolls, hip flexor stretches, mermaid side stretches, child pose, spine twist laying down, cat and cow spinal stretches or calf and hamstring stretches. They will also ease any muscular pain ahead of bedtime.

# QI-BASED PRACTICES: TAI CHI AND QIGONG

The qi (also spelled chi and pronounced "chee"), in traditional and contemporary Chinese culture, is defined as the vital energy that flows in all living entities throughout the universe. It is essential to maintain health and balance, and if it becomes blocked or still then the body becomes weak and unwell, which can lead to sleep deprivation or insomnia.

Tai chi and Qigong (pronounced "chee gong") are ancient Chinese practices that are thought to increase life span by improving health and well-being. Both are based on the qi, combining slow movements with breath and relaxation, but there are differences between the two.

In Qigong, part of traditional Chinese medicine (TCM), you work or train with life energy. It is practiced either moving or motionless for medical purposes, meditative well-being, or as a martial art. Qigong movements are gentle, controlled, graceful, and repetitive, such as oscillating the spine, alternating moving limbs, stretching, and shaking the body or shoulders. It is often labeled as "moving meditation" or "Chinese yoga" and aims to create alignment, coordination, and inner connection.

Qigong exercises are coordinated with breathing through the nose while the mind focuses on the qi flowing through the energetic pathways and meridian points, until the body is fully relaxed.

Qigong is also practiced as motionless meditation and its followers believe it to be more powerful than moving Qigong because its power treats diseases and provides emotional and spiritual healing.

Tai chi is a healing martial art practiced as slow, fluid, continuous movements with specific poses and breathing. If done properly, tai chi can stimulate and free energetic pathways allowing the qi to flow through the body and energize all organs and cells. The art of tai chi is a moving meditation that is considered less intense or profound than meditative Qigong, but tai chi moves are more intricate and more elaborate.

# CROSS-LATERAL MOVEMENTS

Cross-lateral movements, also called cross-crawl or cross-body movements, are intriguing in that they can either calm or energize you. The concept is to connect and coordinate the left and right hemispheres of your brain through coordinated movements, alternating opposites sides of your body, with movements such as marching, crawling, walking, or swimming. The right arm is synched with the left leg, and the left arm is coordinated with the right leg, allowing electrical impulses and information to pass freely between the two parts of your brain, stabilizing your nervous system, creating a relaxed state that makes you feel calm and ready for sleep. An easy cross-lateral exercise is to march gently for 2 to 5 minutes, alternating touching your right knee with your left hand, then your left knee with your right hand.

## MINDFUL WALKING

This mindfulness practice makes you deeply aware of your movements and the sensations in your body as you walk. It is a moving meditation that takes you out of the usual autopilot mode as you focus on the present moment, being aware of your breath and paying close attention to your surroundings as you walk.

## NATURE WALKS

Reconnecting with and absorbing nature might be the most natural thing to do for better sleep. A fascinating Japanese study[3] found that two hours of forest walking on eight different weekend days improved the sleep quality of its participants. Interestingly, walking in the afternoon further extended the length of sleep, compared to walking before noon. Scientists believe that the physiological and psychological benefits of forest walking are due mainly to physical exercise, lowering blood pressure and cortisol levels, thereby reducing stress. Scientists and medical professionals have observed that an environment incorporating natural scenery and green spaces has a beneficial impact on human health, healing, and recovery.

Therapeutic concepts such as "forest bathing" and "ecotherapy" retreats are increasingly popular, and are proven to improve sleep significantly.

## EARTHING OR GROUNDING

Earthing (or grounding) means having direct physical contact with the surface of the Earth, usually by walking barefoot, connected to conductive systems that transfer the Earth's electrons from the ground into the body. The research demonstrates that this may be "a simple, natural, and yet profoundly effective environmental strategy against chronic stress, autonomic nervous system dysfunction, inflammation, pain, poor sleep, and many other ailments including cardiovascular disease".[4] Earthing could be as essential to our well-being as sunshine, clean air and water, nutritious food, and physical activity.

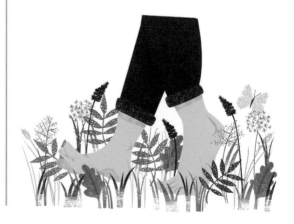

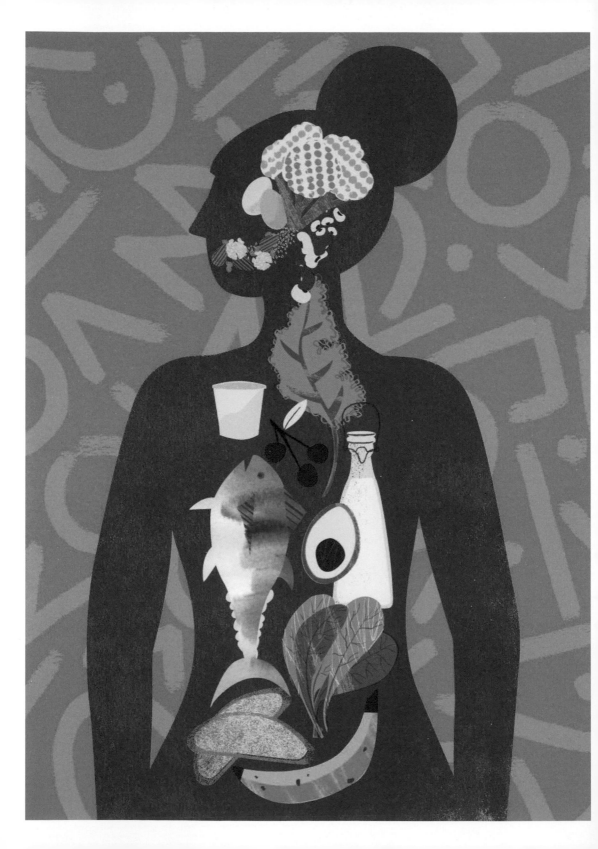

# FEEDING YOUR SLEEP

By understanding the healing power of food, you can make better nutritional choices to improve your sleep. This section provides information and guidance on which foods and nutrients to prioritize and the ones to minimize. Generally speaking, you need to eat a balanced and healthy diet that includes a wide variety of natural whole foods. It is also essential to limit any stimulants especially close to bedtime, and crucial to eat reasonable amounts of food at regular times, every single day. Bear in mind that we are all different and our bodies and brains can respond differently to food choices, so it is important to experiment, observe your reactions, and consult a nutritionist. Of course, always avoid foods that cause allergies or intolerances.

## LESS SLEEP MEANS EATING MORE

When we are sleep deprived or if we don't get good-quality sleep, we subconsciously make worse eating decisions and eat more. We are very likely to struggle to respect regular eating times.

The region of the brain that regulates how much food and the type of food you eat is influenced by the quality and duration of your sleep. Ghrelin, the hunger and appetite hormone, is stimulated by sleep deprivation and, as a result, our brain signals to us that we should go on a hunt for food to build more energy. Meanwhile leptin, the hunger suppression hormone that lets us know when we are full and satisfied, is inhibited. This can happen after a single night of poor sleep. Being sleep-deprived results in eating more, making poorer and emotionally driven decisions toward sweet, salty, and greasy foods which,

when combined with volume eating, results in weight gain, struggling to lose weight, and, for some, obesity.

Ideally, even when you are exhausted, try to select fiber-rich foods that are low in calories, but still filling, such as vegetables, fruits, whole grains, beans, lean meats, and oily fish to support your sleep.

## EATING BEFORE BEDTIME

We need to manage our food intake wisely before going to sleep. Eating heavy, greasy, acidic, or spicy meals before bedtime is likely to lead to a restless night's sleep, and more so if they are foods you are not used to consuming.

When we sleep, our digestion slows down, so eating more food than we can digest can cause sleep disruption and discomfort. We are wired to hunt and eat in the daytime and recuperate overnight. Eating large meals during late hours sends a confusing signal to the brain that it might be hunting time. This results in a boost to our metabolism and a raised body temperature, which lowers our ability to sleep since our core body temperature is meant to dip before going to sleep.

If you are not used to eating spicy food, it can cause indigestion, heartburn, acid reflux, and elevate your core body temperature.

For some people, eating high-protein foods too close to bedtime may disrupt sleep because the body puts more effort into digesting proteins rather than in sleeping.

Try these tips for a better night's sleep:

+ Eat your evening meal a minimum of 2 to 4 hours before bedtime.
+ Avoid eating large meals in the evening, especially heavy, greasy, acidic, and spicy foods if you're not used to them.
+ Prioritize foods rich in tryptophan (see page 111), the serotonin precursor.
+ Avoid fast-release carbohydrates and include some slow-release complex carbohydrates.
+ Avoid tyrosine-rich foods (see page 117) in the evening if you are sensitive to it.
+ Be careful with citrus fruits before bedtime as their acidity can cause heartburn, keeping you up at night.

# EAT TOO LITTLE? STRUGGLE TO SLEEP

While eating too much or the wrong foods in the evening can prevent us from sleeping soundly, eating too little can also have a negative effect because we need enough energy while we sleep to support all the physical, mental, cleansing, growth, and repair processes that take place overnight. Not eating enough calories can cause us to wake up several times during the night, instead of lasting until breakfast. Also see the hypoglycemia section on page 110 for more information.

# DIETARY STRATEGY FOR IMPROVED SLEEP

Try these dietary tips to help you sleep better:

+ Eat regularly—three main meals and two snacks daily.
+ Avoid going longer than 4 to 5 hours without eating. If fasting (see opposite), make sure to eat sufficiently during eating periods.
+ Have a protein-rich breakfast within 45 minutes of awakening.
+ Include a rich source of protein (30 percent), vegetables, fiber, and complex carbohydrates in your meals.
+ Combine protein foods rich in the amino acid tryptophan (see page 111) with low glycemic index

# DETOX OR INTERMITTENT FASTING

Alternating small periods of eating with long periods of not eating, with diets such as intermittent fasting and detox, is gaining in popularity for enhancing health, mental clarity, performance, and fat loss. Research showed that a 1-week fasting period promoted the subjective quality of sleep as well as daytime performance in non-obese people. It showed a fasting-induced increase in the quality of sleep, daytime concentration, energy, and emotional balance.[1]

An intermittent fasting schedule can possibly have a positive effect on your circadian rhythm by regulating daily hormone fluctuations and improving the balance between rapid eye movement (REM) sleep and non-REM sleep, with fewer awakenings throughout the night.

That said, if you do not eat sufficiently during the allowed eating windows, fasting for prolonged periods of time can result in an exaggerated release of the stress hormone cortisol, and accumulating too much cortisol throughout the day can prevent you from falling or staying asleep at night.

So if you follow a fasting diet, make sure you eat sufficiently and that your meals include one-third of protein and two-thirds complex carbohydrates and vegetables to have a more restful sleep.

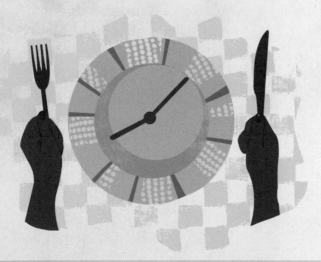

Caution: Fasting might not be advisable for you if you are feeling stressed or anxious, because calorie restriction may increase your cortisol levels and worsen your sleep.

carbohydrate foods (slow-release complex carbohydrate), especially at dinnertime.

+ Limit caffeine to 1 to 2 cups a day (depending on your sensitivity to caffeine) and consume before 2 pm.
+ Ideally, eliminate alcohol completely (see pages 107–108) until your sleep settles.
+ Minimize fermented, acidic, and spicy foods in the evening, if you are not used to eating them.
+ Drink mostly during the day—enough water to urinate 5 to 8 times a day.
+ Stop drinking a minimum of 1.5 to 2 hours before bedtime.

+ Eat at least 5 to 7 portions of fruit and vegetables daily.
+ Eat at least one portion of leafy greens daily.
+ Eat a handful of nuts/dried fruits/seeds twice a day, ideally as snacks.
+ Add a quarter teaspoon of cinnamon to a drink, oatmeal, or yogurt to ease sugar cravings.
+ If you do wake up because of hunger, eat a sleep-friendly snack (see page 112 for suggestions).
+ Get out into the sunlight for at least 30 minutes a day during the brightest part of the day for natural vitamin D production, even if it is cloudy outside (use SPF skin protection).
+ If you feel genuinely hungry before bedtime or know that you easily have overnight blood sugar drops, eat one last small snack 30 minutes before bedtime—it should be light with a combination of protein, complex carbohydrates, and sleep-inducing tryptophan ingredients and magnesium.

## THE ANTI-SNORING NUTRITIONAL STRATEGY

To help minimize snoring, avoid alcohol, as it is a strong muscle relaxant that weakens your respiratory system while you sleep. Avoid oranges and dairy products to prevent the forming of mucus in the airways. Try inhaling eucalyptus or consuming licorice, ginger, or peppermint to clear the respiratory airways.

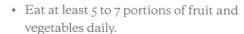

# TRUSTING YOUR GUT

Expressions of stress, fear, anxiety, excitement, and intuition can be manifested with and through our gut, which is often referred to as our "second brain." The gut strangely resembles the brain, with its own nervous system and neurotransmitters. The human intestinal microbiome (the collection of microorganisms such as bacteria and fungi) has an incredible role in sending signals throughout the body and the brain. It plays an important role in our sleep-wake cycle and stress levels among many other functions. And many signals are sent from the gut to the brain along the vagus nerve, which runs internally from the abdomen to the base of the brain. Interestingly, this nerve also serves as the off switch helping relaxation and muscle tension release.

What's more, 90-95 percent of serotonin, the calming and happiness hormone and sleep neurotransmitter, is synthesized in the gut. Friendly bacteria in the digestive tract use the amino acid tryptophan, present in certain foods we eat (see page 111), to produce serotonin. At nighttime, serotonin undergoes two metabolic changes to become melatonin, the hormone that induces and promotes good sleep and generally helps regulate our circadian rhythm. Decreased serotonin levels can lead to anxiety, depression, and increased cravings for carbohydrate foods.

Eating tryptophan-rich foods, especially at dinnertime, is a safe and effective option to boost melatonin and improve your sleep and your mood without unwanted side effects. Our body does not create tryptophan, which is why we have to absorb it from the food we eat. Results will be even more efficient when supplementing tryptophan-rich foods with magnesium, folic acid, zinc, and vitamin B6, or a B-complex.

# SLEEP ENEMIES

You will have heard it over and over—avoid stimulants such as caffeine, alcohol, sugar, and drugs, especially close to bedtime. Stimulants are great to give you a boost and make you feel awake, alert, or focus temporarily, but often interfere with the overall sleep cycles and cause ups and downs, for example having fluctuating moods and energy levels, leading to unhealthy sleep patterns. Let's look into this a little closer.

## ALCOHOL

Alcohol is an effective sedative, making you feel relaxed and drowsy, and it will put you to sleep fast, but if consumed in large amounts, it is guaranteed to cause you to wake up 3 to 4 hours after sleep onset and to disrupt your sleep cycle, in particular REM sleep. You should aim to avoid alcohol consumption, or at least limit it depending on your sensitivity level, following medical guidelines, and have your last alcoholic drink at least 5 hours before bedtime so it doesn't interfere with your sleep quality. Here are some reasons why alcohol affects your sleep:

+ Worryingly, alcohol slows the clearance of adrenaline by the liver and blocks the turning off of adrenaline.
+ Dehydration from drinking too much alcohol keeps your brain on alert.

- You are more likely to snore after drinking, which can impact your sleep.
- You are more likely to wake up because you need to go to the bathroom.
- Unreasonable alcohol consumption will disrupt serotonin levels in the brain, which impacts on sleep and will worsen anxiety, especially as the effects of alcohol wear off.
- Alcohol has a stimulating effect once it metabolizes, so drinking alcohol less than 5 hours before bedtime is likely to disrupt your sleep.

## CAFFEINE

Caffeine is a well-known central nervous stimulant and contained in a wide range of foods and products. Used in the morning or throughout the day for a boost of energy, it triggers the release of adrenaline, giving us strength and focus while switching on our survival mode. The extent to which the effects will be felt depend on your sensitivity level. Caffeine binds to adenosine receptors in the brain, blocking their ability to signal us when we feel sleepy. It can interfere

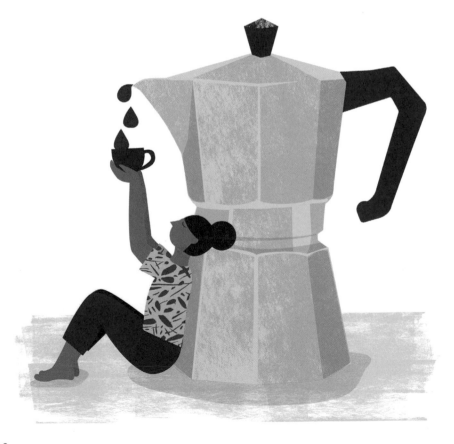

with sleep by keeping your mind alert and overactive. Common side effects are a rapid and irregular heart rate, feeling dizzy and light-headed, anxiety, dehydration, and insomnia.

It can take from 5 to 8 hours to metabolize caffeine, so if you'd like to improve your sleep, limit your consumption drastically and allow an 8-hour window between your last cup of coffee and your bedtime. It may take up to 10 days to go through the withdrawal stage, symptoms of which are headaches and fatigue. If you really must have your cup of coffee, try to limit consumption to one or two cups a day, no later than 2 pm.

Ideally limit or avoid the following until your sleep is back to normal:

+ Coffee, decaffeinated coffee (this still contains some caffeine), mocha.
+ Cacao, chocolate, hot chocolate: The darker the chocolate, the higher the level of the cocoa, the more caffeine there will be, although the amounts are lower than in coffee.
+ Black tea, iced tea, decaffeinated tea, green tea, but the caffeine amounts are much lower than in coffee.
+ Energy and soda drinks that are high in caffeine and sugar.
+ Guarana, yerba mate, acai, and matcha, depending on how sensitive you are.
+ Prescription and non-prescription drugs, if they contain caffeine, but always seek medical advice before stopping any medication.

If you need support with caffeine withdrawal:

+ Reduce your coffee intake by a half-cup a day, gradually decreasing over the week.
+ Take caffeine-free painkillers for the headaches only as needed.
+ Go on brisk walks to stay alert.
+ Try Swiss Water® decaffeinated coffee, which is 99.9 percent caffeine-free.
+ Exercise regularly to boost your energy levels.
+ Sip energizing herbal teas such as matcha (green tea leaves) as a milder alternative. It contains much less caffeine than coffee and it contains the amino acid L-theanine (see page 114), which keeps the mind relaxed and focused. It is a great energy booster to start your day and it contains lots of antioxidants, too.

## NICOTINE-BASED PRODUCTS

Nicotine-based products, cigarettes, or e-cigarettes can interfere with sleep. Research conducted by the Department of Psychology of the University of Wisconsin–Madison[2] showed that smoking was associated with difficulty initiating sleep and waking up, daytime sleepiness, and nightmares, resulting in sleep fragmentation and psychological disturbance. The sooner you can quit smoking, the faster you will find your way to a good night's sleep.

# PHYSIOLOGICAL FACTORS

## ADRENAL DYSFUNCTION (ADRENAL FATIGUE)

Although not widely recognized by the medical and scientific profession, most complementary and alternative medicine practitioners believe that adrenal fatigue exists. It is thought to be caused by an overstimulation of the adrenal glands and a depletion of cortisol and adrenaline reserves as a consequence of being stressed psychologically and physiologically. The adrenal depletion causes brain fog, low energy, depressive mood, salt and sweet cravings, and light-headedness. This condition can be measured by completing an adrenal stress index test. If confirmed, this condition can be supported with a selection of foods, supplemental nutrients, and herbs which can help you get back on the path to good sleep. Please refer to one of the many books on this complex subject.

## BLOOD-SUGAR IMBALANCE

To sleep well, it is essential to keep your blood-sugar levels stable and avoid fluctuating insulin and energy levels that will result in poor sleep and mood changes. Elevated blood sugar boosts insulin levels, making the blood sugar then drop, which triggers a sharp release of cortisol, which in turn prompts the need to eat more sugary foods. This vicious circle, called reactive hypoglycemia, is often caused by insufficient amounts of protein, fiber, and good fats, an excess of sugars and/or fast-release carbohydrates, and causes biological stress possibly leading to insomnia. As a result, stress hormones like adrenaline and cortisol might surge during the night, which will make it harder to fall or stay asleep. You might wake up in the early hours of the night, with your heart racing.

Cortisol levels should be very low when you go to bed and only start rising gradually closer to wake-up time and reach its peak in the first part of the day. But if your blood sugars are not balanced, or you've not eaten sufficiently during the day, cortisol levels will already be too high when you go to bed. This also means you're likely to be up way earlier than desired.

You may notice symptoms of hypoglycemia if you feel moody, easily irritated, anxious, dizzy, and agitated. If you experience this, it is most important to eat regularly. The food ratio for each of your meals should be approximately 30 percent proteins and 70 percent carbohydrates and vegetables combined to prepare the body and brain to sleep. Too much protein, however, will signal the brain to produce dopamine, which is a stimulating rather than a relaxing hormone.

# SLEEP FRIENDS

Nutrients can be grouped into six categories: Carbohydrate, protein, lipid (fat), water, vitamins, and minerals. Foods naturally packed with essential vitamins and minerals can help you prepare for a good night's sleep, especially when eaten at certain times of the day. You can also get these nutrients as over-the-counter dietary supplements, but it is recommended to absorb them from the foods you eat instead if you can.

## TRYPTOPHAN-RICH FOODS: THE SEROTONIN PRECURSORS

It is recommended you eat at least three of these food categories, especially for dinner:

+ **MEATS**: Turkey, steak, chicken, lamb
+ **SEAFOOD/FISH**: Salmon, tuna, sardines, halibut, shrimp, cod
+ **VEGETABLES**: Tomatoes, asparagus, cauliflower, cucumber, celery, cabbage, onions
+ **GREENS**: Broccoli, Swiss chard, green beans, Brussels sprouts, lettuce, spinach, green peas, collard greens, turnip greens
+ **NUTS**: Almonds, peanuts, walnuts, cashews
+ **SEEDS**: Pumpkin, sunflower, sesame, flaxseed

+ **LEGUMES**: Lentils, black beans, kidney beans, chickpeas
+ **DAIRY**: Milk, yogurt, cottage cheese, eggs
+ **GRAINS**: Oats, brown rice, quinoa, wheat
+ **CARBOHYDRATES**: Potatoes in their skins, sweet potato, pasta, wholemeal pasta
+ **BREADS**: Rye bread, wholemeal bread
+ **FRUITS**: Banana, kiwi, dates, apricot

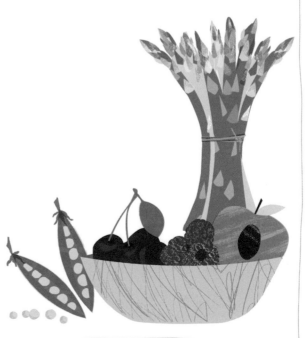

This is an example dietary strategy for blood-sugar imbalance:

+ Eat little and often (six smaller meals) with snacks mid-morning, mid-afternoon, and before bedtime, to avoid cravings and stress hormones spikes.
+ Always include protein, fibrous foods, complex carbohydrates, and low glycemic index foods (labeled low GI), and stay away from sugary foods and drinks.
+ Eat your last snack 30 minutes before bedtime. It should be light with a combination of protein, complex carbohydrates, and sleep-inducing tryptophan and magnesium. For example, a bowl of fortified cereal and milk, a light turkey sandwich, your favorite nut butter on toast, cheese with seeded oat crackers, yogurt with a spoon of honey, rye bread with cottage cheese, a half banana with a tablespoon of nut butter, or a handful of nuts and dried fruit.

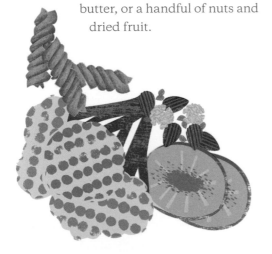

+ Eat your breakfast within 45 minutes of waking up.
+ Add a quarter teaspoon of cinnamon to a drink, oatmeal, or yogurt to ease sugar cravings.
+ Avoid or minimize soft (sugary) drinks, alcoholic drinks, cookies, cakes, and candy.

## VITAMINS

**VITAMIN B5 (pantothenic acid):** Helps with early awakening, depression, irritability, and sleep disorders. Can be found in meat (pork, chicken, turkey, duck, beef, liver, and kidneys), fish (salmon, lobster, and shellfish), whole-grain breads and cereals, dairy products (eggs, milk, yogurt, and milk products), legumes (lentils, split peas, soybeans), vegetables (mushrooms, avocado, broccoli, sweet potatoes, corn, cauliflower, kale, and tomatoes).

**VITAMIN B6:** Helps convert tryptophan into melatonin. A deficiency in B6 is also linked to symptoms of depression and mood disorders, which can lead to insomnia. You can find it in flaxseed, sunflower seeds, pistachios, fish (salmon, tuna, halibut), meat (chicken, pork, beef, turkey), eggs, milk, chickpeas, banana, avocado, and spinach.

**VITAMIN D3:** Lifts the mood, supports sleep, and is essential for the production of serotonin and melatonin. After it is consumed in the diet or absorbed (synthesized) in the skin with sunlight, vitamin D is transported to the liver and kidneys where it is converted to its active hormone form. Seasonal affective disorder (SAD) and a deficiency in vitamin D3 have been linked to sleep issues. SAD can also be corrected with exposure to daylight or specialist lamps (see pages 69-70). Vitamin D can be found in salmon, herring, sardines, cod liver oil, canned tuna, mushrooms, liver, and egg yolk.

## DIETARY MINERALS AND OTHER NUTRIENTS

### MAGNESIUM GLYCINATE

People with low magnesium often experience restless sleep, overnight leg cramps, restless legs, and waking up frequently during the night. Magnesium glycinate, in particular, facilitates restorative sleep and tension release. If you experience frequent muscle tension and back pain, you may have magnesium deficiency. Magnesium glycinate helps calm the nervous system, relieve anxiety, and reduce the stress hormone cortisol. Include a magnesium supplement in your diet and complement it with magnesium bath soaks. It is also best to combine magnesium glycinate with vitamin B6, vitamin C, and calcium for best results.

Excellent sources of magnesium are:

+ Vegetables: Broccoli, dark leafy greens (baby spinach, kale, collard greens)
+ Legumes, whole grains, and soybeans
+ Nuts and seeds: Almonds, Brazil nuts, cashews, pine nuts, flaxseed, sunflower seeds, pecans
+ Fish: Salmon, halibut, tuna, mackerel
+ Fruits: Banana, avocado
+ Dairy: Milk and other dairy products

### CALCIUM

Calcium deficiency can cause you to wake up in the middle of the night and have difficulty returning to sleep. Calcium helps the brain use tryptophan to manufacture the sleep-inducing hormone melatonin (see pages 22-24). Dairy products (milk-based products) contain both tryptophan and calcium, and are some of the best sleep-inducing foods but not the only ones.

Excellent sources of calcium are:

+ Broccoli, dark leafy greens, snap peas
+ Milk, cheese, yogurt
+ Sardines

CAUTION: Note that magnesium glycinate is not to be confused with magnesium citrate, which has a laxative effect. Check with your doctor before taking magnesium supplements as magnesium can interact with medication, and too much of it can cause serious health issues.

+ Fortified cereals
+ Soybeans

## CHROMIUM

Chromium seems to keep blood sugar in balance and can help with cravings. It is an essential nutrient required for sugar and fat metabolism and can be found in broccoli, grape juice, turkey, potatoes, garlic, whole grains, and beef.

## L-THEANINE

This amino acid is found in green tea leaves and helps reduce mental and physical stress. It induces the feeling of calmness, and research shows that it can help reduce psychological stress responses. Japanese researchers showed that L-theanine can improve the quality of your sleep.[3]

## OMEGA-3 FATTY ACIDS

These are one of the "good" types of fat. By facilitating neurotransmitter receptor sensitivity, they have been scientifically proven to improve sleep quality and duration in adults and children in research conducted in the UK, Japan, and Norway. Studies suggest that omega-3 fatty acids from regularly consuming fish may boost your sleep by helping you fall asleep more quickly and improve your daytime performance.[4] Omega-3 is found in rapeseed oil and oily fish such as salmon, mackerel, tuna, sardines, eel, whitebait, and herring.

## MELATONIN

As an over-the-counter or prescribed supplement melatonin should not be used regularly. In the best case scenario, it can sometimes help with jet lag or short-term insomnia, although it might not be as effective as expected in the medium to long term. In the worst case it may disrupt your own natural melatonin production (see pages 22–24). Melatonin supplements are mainly recommended for adults aged 55 or over, to help with short-term sleep problems. There are a few natural dietary sources for melatonin, which might be a better option: Eggs, fish, tart cherries (Montmorency—see opposite), nuts such as almonds and walnuts, berries such as raspberries and goji berries.

# LIQUID SLEEP

Water and hydration are the foundation of good health and well-being. Sleep is no exception to this. It is all about having the right types of liquids and the right level of hydration at the right time of the day, otherwise your sleep could be impacted. Follow these tips for a better night's sleep:

+ Avoid dehydration at all costs. Staying hydrated is a vital human need, and consuming insufficient fluid will create physiological stress and a sense of panic, since your brain will interpret a lack of fluids as a danger. Dehydration also causes headaches, which can disturb your sleep. The general recommendation is to drink 4 to 8 tall glasses of water a day and more if you feel thirsty, with the aim to go to the toilet between 5 to 8 times a day. This will depend on your physical condition, your age, weight, level of activity, and your individual physiological needs, and it is also weather-dependent. Don't forget we all sweat during sleep and lose 16 fl oz of water a night through perspiration.

+ Avoid nighttime bathroom trips that will disrupt your sleep by consuming your last liquids 1.5 to 2 hours before bedtime, so you are able to empty your bladder before going to bed. The same goes for foods with a high water content and diuretics such as watermelon and celery.

+ If you must have alcohol, have your last drink at least 5 hours before bedtime.
+ If you feel thirsty during the night, drink just a few sips of water at a time from a glass at your bedside table.
+ If you are after a comforting sleepy drink as part of your bedtime routine, try an herbal infusion (see page 163).

Here are some suggestions for "sleepy" drinks:

## MONTMORENCY TART CHERRY JUICE

This can also be found in concentrated format to be diluted. It is one of the richest natural sources of melatonin. In 2010, the *Journal of Medicinal Food* found that drinking about 16 fl oz of tart cherry juice during the day could result in a significant increase in sleep duration and decrease in insomnia.

## BANANA TEA

Bananas contain potassium and magnesium, the latter being sleep-inducing. Banana peels have the most concentration of these minerals; therefore banana advocates recommend boiling the banana (peel and fruit) and drinking the banana water itself with a bit of cinnamon. Keep the fruit to use in a smoothie or for dessert!

## PURE COCONUT WATER

Coconut water is often used for reenergizing and rehydration, but it contains ingredients such as magnesium and potassium and vitamin B, which are all excellent for improving your sleep.

## MOON MILKS

Drinking warm milk before bedtime for a good night's sleep is a tradition in many cultures. Milk does not have scientifically proven anti-insomnia properties, but it does contain a small amount of the amino acid tryptophan, which we know is the precursor to serotonin, an essential and natural sleep chemical. If you find drinking warm milk comforting, and a good part of your sleep ritual, there is no harm in having it—it can be a soothing signal to the brain that bedtime is near. Try supplementing your warm milk with healing herbs, wonderful flavors, and sleep-inducing substances such as turmeric (curcuma), rose water, cardamom, ashwagandha powder, honey, or agave syrup. Almond or oat milks are great alternatives if you are lactose intolerant. Many delicious moon milk recipes are widely available online. My favorite one is warm oat or almond milk, mixed with a generous pinch of turmeric, a teaspoon of rosewater, and honey or agave nectar to taste. Make sure you drink your moon milk at least 1.5 to 2 hours before bedtime to avoid bathroom visits during the night.

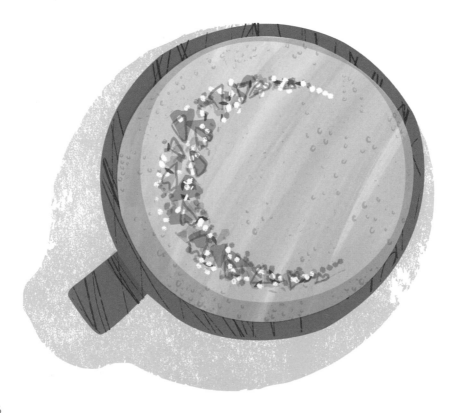

# TYROSINE

Tyrosine is the precursor to dopamine and helps make adrenaline and noradrenaline, the hormones that stimulate your brain and increase vigilance, alertness, attention, and focus. They prepare the body to "fight" or "flee" from a perceived attack. This can increase stress levels and slow down the process of falling asleep. If you realize you are sensitive to it, you should avoid foods containing tyrosine after 5 pm. It is found in foods like chicken, turkey, cheese, tofu, milk, beans, beef, pork, fish (salmon), seeds, nuts, and whole grains, and to a lesser degree in canned tuna, eggs, sweet potatoes, and spinach. However, most of these foods also contain natural sleep-inducing elements, so experiment for yourself or seek professional advice to make the right decision.

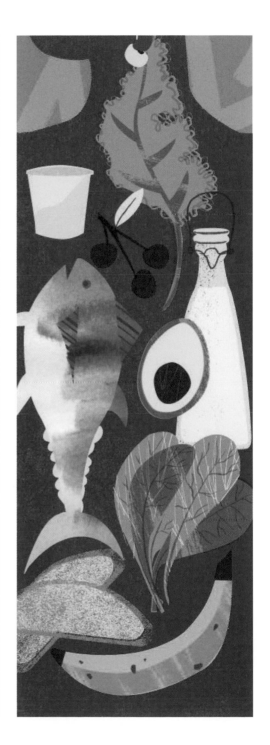

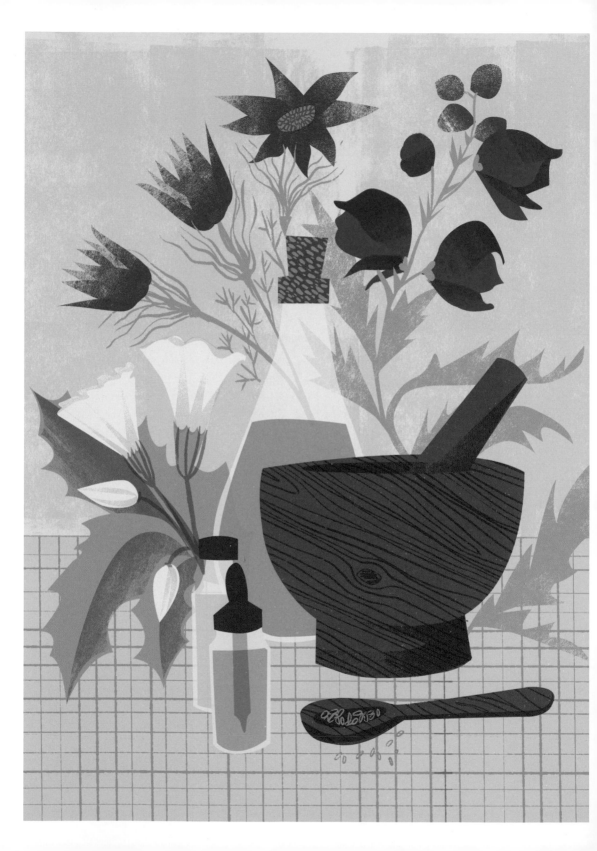

# COMPLEMENTARY AND ALTERNATIVE THERAPIES

When it comes to improving your sleep, it is worth considering complementary and alternative therapies, which can be used as a replacement or in addition to conventional medicine, to restore balance, strength, energy, performance, vitality, and, of course, the sleep we need to repair and support our bodies and our minds. There is a wide range of remedies, treatments, and techniques to choose from, many of which are based on ancient and holistic medicinal systems.

## CAM THERAPIES AND WHEN TO USE THEM

Complementary and alternative medicine (CAM) is designed to improve physical and mental health. It is usually based on naturopathic or energetic theories, which assert that ailments and diseases can be prevented or treated without the use of pharmaceutical drugs or surgery and instead they promote the use of natural elements and products, mind-body based techniques, and physical manipulations.

On the one hand, conventional drugs have been tested by medical and scientific experts in controlled clinical studies before being officially authorized for sale, while natural therapeutic and medicinal products may not have been as rigorously researched to confirm their properties or side effects. That said, most of these therapies have been observed, and tried and tested empirically over time to prove their effectiveness, for 50–5,000 years depending on the therapy.

CAM may be a good option if conventional medical treatments haven't worked for you, if you are experiencing negative side effects, or if you just wish to try a more natural approach. It may also be more affordable to go "natural." You may need to try a range of different therapies before finding which is the right one for you.

## CAM THERAPIES FOR SLEEP

In this section you will find out how the following natural therapies can help you

---

*CAUTION: Before undertaking a new therapy and consulting with a trained CAM professional and/or accredited practitioner, seek medical advice from your doctor to make sure there are no contraindications in your case.*

sleep: Ayurveda, homeopathy, traditional Chinese medicine, body-based therapies, water-based therapies, energy-healing therapies, and contact-based therapies.

In addition, the following therapies, which are also considered complementary or alternative, are explained in their own dedicated sections:

+ Aromatherapy (see pages 170-175)
+ Autogenic therapy (see pages 93-94)
+ Light therapy (see pages 69-71)
+ Herbal medicine (see pages 161-169)
+ Hypnotherapy (see pages 92-93)
+ Meditation (see page 78)
+ Mindfulness (see page 78)
+ Nutritional healing (see pages 103-117)
+ Sophrology (see page 94)
+ Sound therapy (see pages 149-159)
+ Yoga nidra (see page 75)

When reading about each of these natural therapies, keep in mind that the focus for this book is the treatment of sleep issues and insomnia specifically, rather than a complete list of the ailments they can treat.

# AYURVEDA

Ayurveda, a traditional and holistic (whole body and mind) medicinal system, originated in India over 5,000 years ago, making it one of the oldest medicines. It aims to strengthen physical health, but also support emotional,

psychological, and spiritual well-being, by investigating imbalances and making therapeutic recommendations based on individual health profiles. Ayurveda means the "knowledge of life."

According to Ayurveda, sleep issues are caused by an imbalanced "prana vata" ("vata" is our energy through mind and body). Prana vata governs the senses, creativity, breathing, and reasoning. An imbalance can lead to an overactive and worrying mind, difficulties breathing, insomnia, and other sleep issues. Each Ayurvedic health profile is a combination of three "doshas" (also referred to as body types or bioenergies)—vata, pitta, and kapha—which reflect our individual nature in terms of health, body, natural preferences, and personality.

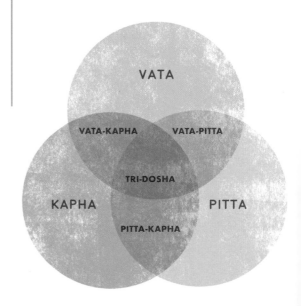

The three doshas are each a different combination of the five basic elements—earth, water, fire, ether (or space), and air. Every individual is conceived with a different combination of the three doshas, but in general one is dominant. Therefore, each person requires their own tailored Ayurvedic recommendations in terms of diet, exercise, treatments, and sleep regime, to keep the three doshas in balance.

**VATA DOSHA** is related to air and space and linked to movement, energy, and creativity. Vata-dominant people tend to have overactive minds, and be restless, worried, and indecisive, which can often make it hard for them to sleep peacefully and deeply. They should follow a nightly wind-down routine (see pages 41-51) and attempt to tame their mind as best as they can (see pages 87-95).

**PITTA DOSHA** is related to fire and water and linked to all metabolic processes. Pitta-dominant people are ambitious, emotional, competitive, and overachievers, which makes their lives perhaps too stressed or too busy to build in enough quiet time, sleep, and rest. Their body temperature is likely to increase more easily, making it more difficult to fall or stay asleep. They should avoid an excess of stimulating activity, bright lighting, or starting a project too close to bedtime. Cooling down the bedroom by opening windows ahead of sleep can also be helpful.

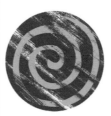

**KAPHA DOSHA** is related to water and earth and linked to some of the liquids and fluids in our bodies. Kapha is referred to as the building blocks representing stability in the body. An overproduction of mucus, for example, is kapha in excess. Kapha people are calm, easygoing, love to eat, and are perhaps sluggish. They also tend not to feel entirely recovered even after a full night's sleep, which means they can be often lethargic, groggy, tired, and sleepy. After ruling out any medical condition that could cause poor sleep quality such as apnea, poor digestion, pain, or nutritional deficiencies, kapha people should follow a regular sleep-wake routine and engage in energizing outdoor activities in the daytime.

## AYURVEDIC TREATMENTS

Ayurveda focuses on the cause and prevention, rather than cure, of diseases and health issues. Its main principle is that wellness depends on the delicate balance between body, mind, and spirit. Often, Ayurvedic treatments include medicinal herbs, spiritual practices such as yoga, meditation, chanting, prayers, and purification ceremonies, therapeutic practices such as detox, breathwork, cleansing, and nature walks, body treatments such as massages, oil treatments, and the activation of specific pressure points.

Ayurvedic medicine relies on a specific diagnostic approach toward a personalized wellness program based on each person's individual mix of doshas, so it is best to consult with a professional Ayurvedic practitioner to design the best healing plan for you. Ayurveda experts will often link sleep issues with other underlying physical or mental health problems, which can be resolved with specific recommendations in terms of diet and lifestyle.

Other interesting aspects of Ayurveda worth exploring to balance doshas, prana vata, and improve your sleep: Mudras hand gestures (see page 80), marma points therapy (see below), and Ayurvedic herbal remedies (see pages 125-126), all of which are also part of this ancient holistic therapeutic system.

## MARMA POINTS THERAPY

According to Ayurveda, the body has 108 marma points—one in the mind and 107 on the body, located on the head, face, arms, legs, chest, torso, abdomen, and back, and at the intersections of veins, ligaments, joints, muscles, nerves, tendons, and bones. Marma points are often referred to as the link between matter and consciousness. According to Vedic principles and wisdom, there are 72,000 energetic channels, also referred to as "nadis," circulating freely throughout the body. Marma points are the points where life force (prana) enters the body and exits the nadis. In other words, they connect the body's energy and life force to the physical self. Health issues can block the energy from flowing freely through marma points and disrupt natural processes or healing, which can lead to poor sleep (amongst other symptoms).

Stimulating marma points by touch or with a massage impacts the chakras and the doshas (bioenergies in the body) and has healing properties for organs, glands, joints, and muscles. It supports important bodily processes, including its biochemistry that produces the hormones and neurochemicals we need to heal and feel better. The principles of marma points therapy are similar to acupressure or acupuncture and it also relieves muscle tension, anxiety, inflammation, and hormonal and digestion issues, all of which are intimately linked to insomnia issues and poor sleep. Marma points therapy clears energy blockages and revitalizes the whole body and mind, encouraging deep and restorative sleep.

Herb-infused oils, ghee, and sesame or coconut oil are often used to massage marma points in a circular clockwise motion to stimulate the energy flow or counterclockwise to achieve relaxation and calm. An Ayurvedic healer will determine which points and products to use depending on your dosha type (see page 121) and ailments to be treated.

A trained Ayurvedic professional should ideally perform marma points therapy, but once you are familiar with each point, you can try self-activating marma points for sleep.

## MARMA POINTS FOR SLEEP

To help ease you into a peaceful slumber, it is a good idea to stimulate these sleep-inducing marma points before bedtime or once you are in bed. Try one point at a time, or all of them in sequence, and monitor how your sleep is affected. You may want to use massage oils infused with essential oils (see pages 174–175), such as lavender, bergamot, and jatamansi, to enhance the relaxing and sedative effects of this Ayurvedic self-massage technique. You can apply a tiny drop of essential oil directly onto the skin with the fingertip, but exercise caution as this could result in allergies or adverse skin reactions. It is generally safer to use them diluted (see page 172) and advisable to do a skin patch test first, and of course seek professional advice. It is also not advised to expose your skin to sunlight after applying essential oils, since some of them can on occasion create a photosensitive reaction.

**AJNA OR STHAPANI MARMA:** This point is located slightly above the middle of the eyebrows at the center of the forehead. Press on this "third eye" center with either your ring finger or your thumb or your joint index and middle fingers, with your eyes closed, breathing gently. Massage in small circular motions and focus on finding calm within yourself. Stimulating this marma point brings stability and order in the body and the mind and as it helps to balance emotions and stress, it is highly recommended to alleviate insomnia.

Another way to stimulate this marma is by resting your forehead on the ground with your knees bent, and sitting back on your heels in the "child's pose," which induces deep relaxation and good sleep.

The Ayurvedic oil treatment "shirodhara" is also very efficient in activating the sthapani marma. It is one of the most popular treatments to alleviate insomnia, an overactive mind, stress, and hormonal imbalances. After a face, neck, and scalp massage, a fine and continuous stream of warm oil infused with herbs and essential oils is gently and slowly poured over the forehead, landing on this marma point. It restores calm and balance to the mind and nervous system and improves sleep and memory.

**MŪRDHNI OR ADHIPATI MARMA:** This point is located at the center of the top of the head, on the highest part of the skull. To find it, place your extended hand against your forehead (base of your hand aligned with your eyebrows), then let your fingers relax over and touch the top of your head. The adhipati marma is two joint fingers further from where your middle finger ends, at the top and center of your skull.

Apply pressure on the adhipati marma with your joint index and middle fingers. Massage in small circular motions and let your shoulders drop and neck relax, breathe, and let your active mind calm down. Stimulating this marma point supports melatonin production (see pages 22–24), enhances sleep, and reduces depression.

ŪRDHVA SKANDHA MARMA: This point is located on the top of the shoulder muscle (trapezius), in the middle but slightly behind, at equal distance between the base of the neck and end of the shoulder. Use the opposite hand to massage in circular motions with your index and middle finger while inhaling and exhaling. Repeat on the opposite shoulder. Then return to the first shoulder, and press the point firmly steadily and continuously. Repeat on the opposite shoulder. If it is too tender, release the pressure slightly and breathe in and out. You should feel immediate release, loosening of the shoulders, and a flow of energy. This helps relieve tension, stress, and mental fatigue, calms the mind, and releases stagnant emotions. It helps improve sleep and creates a sense of tranquility as well as relieving pain and stiffness.

PADA KSHIPRA MARMA: First oil the soles of your feet with either coconut oil, ghee, or sesame oil to make the skin smooth and supple. Then apply a drop of jatamansi essential oil (preferably diluted—see page 172) on this point, which is located in the space between the big toe and the second toe. Press firmly on the point and massage in circular motions. Proceed with each foot. The equivalent point exists in the hands at the muscle between the thumb and index finger. This helps release internalized emotions, helping you to feel more serene and calm.

TALAHRUDAYA OR TALAHRIDAYA MARMA: Position your hand with your palm facing upward. Place your thumb on the center of your palm and your index and middle fingers on the top of your hand, as if you are trying to join your fingers and thumb through your hand. Let your fingers curl up naturally. Squeeze firmly, digging the thumb into your palm, then massage in very small circular motions counterclockwise, while inhaling and exhaling deeply. Then continue on clockwise for a little longer. Make sure to relax your shoulders. It might feel slightly sore or tender, which is normal as we build a lot of tension in our hands—apply enough pressure without causing too much pain. Stimulating this point will reduce stress and anxious feelings. The equivalent point exists in our feet, in the middle of the sole, in line with the middle toe.

## ESSENTIAL AYURVEDIC HERBS FOR SLEEP

Ayurvedic treatments will almost always be supplemented by herbal remedies to support the healing and balancing process. When it comes to sleep, the most notable and typical plants used are ashwagandha, brahmi, jatamansi, and cardamom for their calming, relaxing, and balancing properties, but this is not an exhaustive list. These can be consumed as an infusion or in powder form, perhaps mixed into your favorite milk a few hours before bedtime. "Golden milk" prepared with turmeric, herbs, and spices is also a common relaxing warm beverage ahead of bedtime. These herbal remedies can also be inhaled as an essential oil or applied to marma points (see pages 122-124) preferably diluted in a carrier oil to avoid skin reactions. Some are also available as herbal supplements in capsules form. Seek advice from your doctor and Ayurvedic therapist before consuming.

### ASHWAGANDHA *(Withania somnifera)*
Ashwagandha is one of the most essential therapeutic herbs in Ayurveda and probably the best adaptogen (see pages 166-167)—a plant that can increase our resilience and ability to cope with any form of physical, mental, or emotional stress. Ashwagandha is renowned for reducing anxiety, decreasing the levels of the stress hormone cortisol, and easing insomnia at night, while rejuvenating

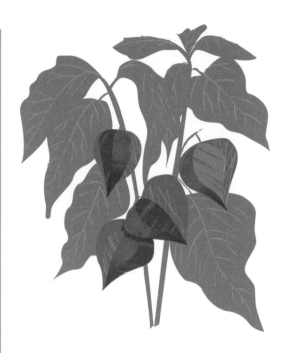

and reenergizing the body during the day, strengthening the nervous system.

A controlled clinical study showed that ashwagandha root extract improved sleep quality, sleep onset, and efficiency in patients with insomnia who were given a dose of 300 mg twice daily.[1] It is generally consumed as a tea or as a powder mixed into warm milk (or milk alternative), soups, smoothies, stews, or other smooth-textured foods, but it can also be taken as capsules or ingested as ashwagandha-infused ghee.

### CARDAMOM *(Elettaria cardamomum)*
Cardamom is a well-known aromatic plant, commonly used as dried pods or seeds, or ground into many Indian dishes, desserts, and in beverages such as chai or warm milks. It belongs to

the same family as ginger and exists in green or black form; the latter being most popular to boost the immune and respiratory systems. In addition to having anti-inflammatory and antibacterial properties, cardamom balances all three doshas (see page 121) bringing internal harmony and a sense of pure well-being. It is calming and helps to relieve anxiety, and is also scientifically proven to have sedative effects.[2] While it can be ingested, inhaling the sweet and soothing aroma of cardamom as an essential oil is perhaps even more efficient to restore the balance of the doshas and induce sleep and relaxation.

### BRAHMI (Bacopa monnieri)

Brahmi is commonly used to treat Alzheimer's disease and other mental illnesses amongst many other ailments, but it is also prescribed for anxiety and depression, calming emotional disorders while supporting concentration and focus and helping with sleep issues including insomnia. It is even more potent when combined with ashwangandha, cardamom, or jatamansi.

### JATAMANSI (Nardostachys jatamansi)

Jatamansi is a member of the valerian (see page 164) family and native of the alpine Himalayas. Also called spikenard, it has insomnia-relieving properties, helping to induce sound and restful sleep with its calming effect, and it treats mental disorders such as anxiety, stress, and depression while rejuvenating the body, mind, and central nervous system. It can be mixed in powder form into an evening hot drink, or inhaled as a few drops of essential oil or diluted into a massage oil, such as jojoba or almond, to stimulate sleep marma points (see pages 123–124). For an enhanced effect, spikenard essential oil blends well with other essential oils such as lemon, geranium, lavender, clary sage, frankincense neroli, rose, patchouli, and vetiver.

## HOMEOPATHY

Homeopathy is a natural alternative approach used for a wide range of health conditions. It was invented in the 18th century by a German doctor named Samuel Hahnemann whose key medicinal theory was that "like cures like," meaning that an agent or substance that causes specific symptoms can also get rid of them and cure the related illness. His second principle was that such substances should be diluted to an infinitesimal dosage making them almost undetectable, yet incredibly potent without being harmful.

Many traditional doctors remain skeptical about homeopathy, thinking it works due to a placebo effect, meaning that the patients heal because they believe in the treatment, rather than due to any properties of the medicine itself. Yet homeopathic remedies do seem to help some people with insomnia and psycho-emotional conditions such as stress, anxiety, and depression, and as a result can help with sleep problems.

## TREATMENT

A typical homeopathic treatment consists of administering micro doses of relevant substances under the tongue either as granules or tablets that dissolve, or as a liquid; they are then absorbed into the bloodstream. Depending on the country and school of thought, practitioners may recommend a "complex" treatment, meaning that it will be a combination of plant, mineral, or animal substances working synergistically at various concentration levels—generally low when treating physical conditions, and higher for emotional and psychological conditions. Other practitioners may prescribe a single remedy at a time to ascertain which is the most effective for you. Homeopathic medicine sold in pharmacies is usually "complex" and contains several agents to treat a specific short-term condition, but is generally not designed to treat long-term ailments. This is why it is always best to consult with a homeopathic practitioner, who can create a personalized holistic treatment plan.

*Note: The single remedies listed below have a wide range of therapeutic indications and the practitioner will adapt them based on your individual assessment: your constitution, prior health issues, your predisposition to certain illnesses, and any current medical issues. Bear in mind that it is possible for your condition to get worse from the treatment before getting better and that children will most likely receive different treatments and dosages than adults.*

## HOMEOPATHIC REMEDIES FOR SLEEP

This is a non-exhaustive list of homeopathic remedies helpful for relaxation and sleep:

+ **ACONITE**: Anxiety, panic attacks
+ **ARGENTUM NITRICUM**: Anxiety, fears, phobias
+ **ARSENICUM ALBUM**: Anxiety, fears from loneliness, self-criticism
+ **CALCAREA CARBONICA**: Anxiety from uncertainty
+ **GELSEMIUM SEMPERVIRENS**: Intense stress, pressure from upcoming event, fear of crowds, fear of public speaking
+ **IGNATIA AMARA**: Sadness, grief, loss, emotional states
+ **KALI ARSENICOSUM**: Fear of death or serious health conditions
+ **KALI PHOPHORICUM**: Night terrors, nightmares, sleepwalking, overwhelming feelings
+ **LYCOPODIUM**: Fear of public speaking, lack of self-confidence

- **PHOSPHORUS:** Anxiety
- **PULSATILLA:** When in need of reassurance and support
- **SILICA:** Fear of the unknown, fear of public speaking or of being the center of attention
- **STRAMONIUM:** Night terrors, nightmares, somber thoughts while awake

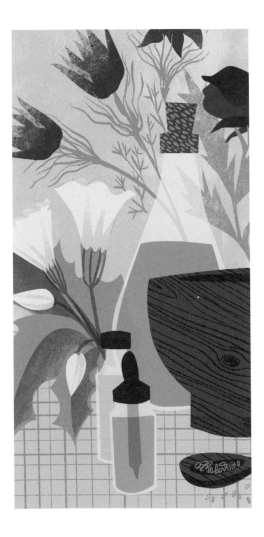

# TRADITIONAL CHINESE MEDICINE

Traditional Chinese medicine (TCM) has been the main medical system used in China for well over 2,000 years and perhaps even up to 3,000 years. Like Ayurveda, TCM is an ancient medicinal approach from Asia relying on holistic principles that are sometimes different than the ones supported by conventional Western medicine. Nevertheless, thousands of years of experimentation and learnings have made it one of the most popular CAM therapies used in the Western world. The aim of TCM is to rebalance our energetic systems, restore our physiological processes, revitalize our organ function, reduce body pain, disorders, and dysfunction, and bring back harmony and wellness into our lives.

The starting point is a diagnostic consultation to gauge your energy levels and assess your overall health by examining the eyes, tongue, skin, and nails, and closely examining the pulse rate—its speed, strength, and any variations. Then proceeding to palpation (touch) and detecting any sounds, breath, and odors emitted by the patient. Detailed questions are then asked to complete the diagnostic.

TCM practitioners target the treatment on affected organs, as this can be the root cause of insomnia. To restore and maintain physical and mental health, TCM treats the mind and body with practices such as acupuncture, Chinese herbal remedies, qi-based practices such as qigong and tai chi (see page 100), tui na (therapeutic massage) cupping, gua sha (a detox method), and nutritional recommendations.

## YIN AND YANG

The yin and yang theory is a fundamental principle of traditional Chinese medicine. Yin and yang are interconnected energies that cannot exist without each other. Opposite yet complementary, together they form a whole and they need to be balanced to restore health and harmony. The internal organs are linked to the yin part of the body, whereas the external aspects of the body are connected to the yang.

## QI

The other TCM fundamental is qi (pronounced "chee") energy, which flows throughout all living things and the whole universe. Qi is the vital life force that runs through the human body's energetic channels, also called meridians. Stagnant or blocked qi will generate illness or disorders in the body.

According to TCM, "wei qi" is a type of qi that has a strong protective energy. It runs on the external yang parts of the body during the daytime while we are awake and active, and at night while we sleep it runs on the internal yin part, to restore our vital organs and replenish our jing and hormones. Jing is the fluid essence in our body that contains the life force and is connected to the growth, repair, and maturation of each individual—it is essential to maintain good health and live a long life.

Someone suffering from chronic insomnia or sleep deprivation won't benefit from this overnight healing process and it will be apparent from the dry and wrinkly appearance of their skin. Similarly strong negative emotions such as anger, stress, and upset feelings will cause the qi to stagnate in the liver, and cause the patient to overeat at nighttime resulting in food being stuck in the stomach. These blockages will prevent wei qi from flowing through the liver and stomach, forcing it to stay outside of the body as opposed to flowing internally as it should. As a result, a patient will struggle to sleep.

Another cause of sleeplessness is if a particular organ is experiencing dampness (an excess of fluid, mucus, or phlegm), is exposed to the cold (caused by external temperature, low metabolism, or cold drinks and foods), or is inhibited by a tumor growth. In such circumstances, wei qi cannot penetrate into the organ, and, as a result, the patient will wake up every night at the same time and struggle to get back to sleep until the TCM body clock shifts to another organ.

# THE TCM BODY CLOCK

According to TCM, each organ has its time of glory around the 24-hour circadian clock. Our energy shifts inward in the hours before midnight (from about 9 pm) to nurture our emotions and our internal organs. Qi energy flows through the body's meridians (or channels) in a 24-hour cycle, processes emotions, and moves from one organ to the next every two hours to cleanse, repair, rebalance, and restore its function one at a time. If we don't sleep during such processes, our organ(s) may become unhealthy over time, and conversely, if an organ is unhealthy, it can cause insomnia at this time. The same applies during the day—if you feel particularly low in energy at a specific time, it might indicate an organ deficiency or imbalance because each function in our body is connected to a precise time on our body clock.

According to TCM, bedtime should be around 10:30 pm with the aim of falling asleep by 11 pm. The time at which you fall asleep is as important as the total duration of sleep you get, if not more so.

**11 pm–1 am, gallbladder function:** Sleep onset, release digestive bile, cell repair. A blockage could be caused by alcohol, fatty or spicy foods, or late-night eating.

**1–3 am, liver function:** Cleanse, blood detox, recovery, deep sleep. A blockage could be caused by a heavy diet, late-night meal, alcohol consumption, or stress.

**3–5 am, lungs function:** Lungs detox, dreams, and memory consolidation. A blockage could be cause by a weak immune system, fatigue, sadness, or anger.

**5–7 am, large intestine:** Bowel release, wake-up time.

## CHINESE HERBAL MEDICINE

Chinese medicinal herbs have been used to treat insomnia for thousands of years. The aim is to rectify the balance and activity of the yin and yang and restore the body to its natural healthy physiological state. TCM doctors prescribe a preparation of several Chinese herbal remedies with sedative, hypnotic, anti-anxiety, and antidepression properties to help treat insomnia.

In 2003, an extensive survey was conducted in Taiwan, Province of China, to look into the usage patterns of over 6,800 patients commonly taking Chinese herbal medicine to help improve insomnia symptoms.[3] The survey showed that most prescriptions were prescribed 3 times a day in synergetic combination. The most frequently prescribed herbal medicine was Jia-Wey-Shiau-Yau-San, which combines *Angelica sinensis*, *Atractylodes macrocephala*, *Paeonia lactiflora*, *Bupleurum chinese*, and *Wolfiporia extensa*. Hong Hua or Safflower (*Carthamus tinctorius*) was also prescribed, but it is mostly used to enhance blood circulation.

Other popular herbal prescriptions for insomnia are Ren Shen Gui Pi Wan (herbal combination formula), Suanzaoren (*Ziziphus spinosa*, as a decoction), and Gancao (*Glycyrrhiza uralensis*). Traditional Chinese medicine remedies such as *Schisandrae Chinensis Fructus*, *Albiziae Flos*, *Polygalae Radix*, *Longan Arillus*, and *Ganoderma* have also

been prescribed for their natural sedative properties. These herbs and formulas are prepared from flowers, stems, stalks, leaves, cork, seeds, and roots. They are either prepared as a decoction (boiled to extract active agents from the plant) then consumed as a hot drink, or taken as pills, tablets, capsules, or tinctures. The treatment duration lasts from a few weeks to a few months. See also the Healing Plants section on pages 161–169.

## ACUPUNCTURE

Acupuncture is a fundamental component of traditional Chinese medicine and probably the best-known TCM treatment in Western culture. It consists of swiftly inserting very fine sterilized single-use needles into specific points on the surface of the skin to stimulate the acupoints located along the meridians (or energetic channels). The practitioner will select the points

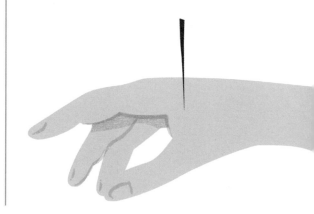

to treat deficient organs, cure specific ailments, alleviate physical pain, and relieve muscle tension. The needles are left in place for 20 to 30 minutes, on average, while the patient rests. The practitioner might wiggle them from time to time to stimulate the nerves and create an energetic shift restoring the qi flow (see page 129). This results in balancing the qi within the body and being fully relaxed, improving sleep, increasing energy levels, and maintaining a serene and balanced mind, which can happen immediately or require several sessions. One research study found that acupuncture was more effective in alleviating insomnia than a commonly prescribed sleeping pill.[4]

## CUPPING TECHNIQUE

Cupping is a TCM technique of placing warm bulb-shaped glass cups on the skin surface. Warming the air inside of the cup before positioning it creates a strong suction, which pulls the skin to improve blood circulation and detoxify the body. The cups are generally placed on the back, neck, and shoulders and gently lifted after a duration determined by the practitioner (usually between 5 to 20 minutes). Another technique involves gliding the warm cups over the back along the meridians. This treatment removes stagnation and stimulates the flow of qi energy (see page 129). A clinical scientific study of patients aged 18-50

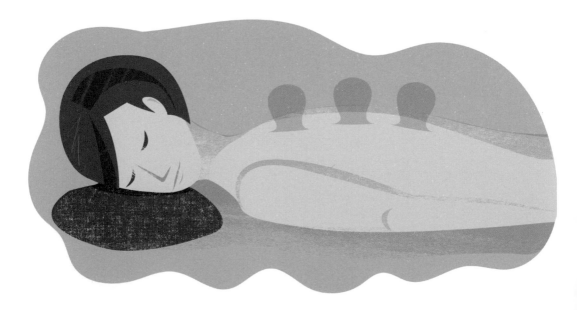

found that cupping effectively reduces pain and restlessness and improves sleep.[5] Cupping may leave bruise-like traces on the body, which fade in a few days. It is not generally considered a harmful treatment, but is perhaps not the most cosmetically pleasing.

## GUA SHA

"Gua sha" (pronounced "gwah shah") is an ancient method facilitating the detoxification of the body and expelling unnecessary and harmful heat. An oily product is rubbed onto the body with a smooth round massage tool used to stroke and scrape the skin energetically on the back, neck, arms, and legs. This type of healing massage moves the blood and lymph at the body's skin surface to break up qi energy (see page 129) stagnation points. Gua sha can have a further impact underneath the skin, reaching deep and soft tissues all the way to the internal organs. It helps improve blood circulation, remove cellular waste, eliminate toxins, and promotes the production of new cells. It has also been scientifically proven to reduce perimenopausal symptoms,[6] which include insomnia, anxiety, sweating, and fatigue. It supports the immune system, reduces inflammation, back pain, tightness, headaches, and regulates energy levels and body temperature. All of these factors can be contributing factors to sleep disruption if they are not managed properly.

## TUI NA

"Tui na" (pronounced "twee-nah") is an essential form of therapeutic massage practiced in TCM, based on the same principles as acupuncture and acupressure, as it works on the system of meridians and acupoints to support and stimulate the flow of qi (see page 129) throughout the body and helps remove any blockages that are causing qi energy to stagnate. It also supports mental and emotional functions. Tui na is often used in combination with acupuncture and follows the same principles of energy balancing. This massage technique is either gentle or energetic, depending on the patient's needs, and can involve stretching and joint loosening. Tui na is recommended to relieve insomnia.

---

CAUTION: Gua sha can cause capillaries (fine vessels near the skin surface) to burst, which can result in light purple or red bruising, called "sha." This disappears after a few days.

## ACUPRESSURE

Acupressure, tui na, and acupuncture are all based on the principle of removing stagnating qi (see page 129), which causes pain, insomnia, psychological problems, and many health issues. Acupressure is often considered to be needle-free acupuncture. The practitioner applies gentle yet firm pressure with their hands and fingers, but also elbows or feet sometimes, generally on a fully clothed patient. Each acupoint is worked on from a few seconds to a few minutes in circular motions along the meridian channels, which helps restore the energy flow and balance of key internal organs. As a result, it can also help ease symptoms of insomnia. This can be done by a practitioner or performed at home by yourself once you know the precise location of each acupressure point.

Note that the points are the same for acupressure and acupuncture.

+ The most popular acupoint for sleep is called "an mian," located on the two protruding bones in the back of the head, behind your ears on each side in the hollow grooves where the skull meets the neck. Massaging the an mian points will induce sleep and reduce stress, anxiety, headaches, and migraines.

+ Another insomnia-relieving acupressure point is the wrist's "shen men," positioned in the inside of the wrist on the external side closest to the little finger. A study showed that a 5-week acupressure treatment on this acupoint on each side relieved insomnia symptoms.[7]

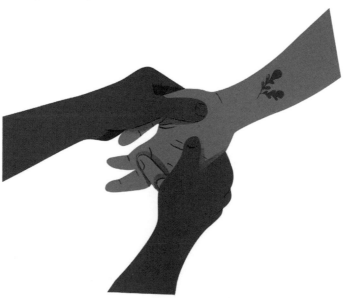

+ A third acupoint called "tai chong" is commonly used to alleviate stress, anxiety, sleeplessness, and insomnia. It is located on the very top of the foot at the junction of the big toe and the second toe's metatarsals. Another closely related tai chong point is in the same line but slightly lower, closer to the first and second toes junction.

+ Another excellent acupoint for sleep is "yin tang," located in the center of the forehead between the eyebrows above the start of the nose. It is often activated to relieve insomnia, anxiety, agitation, headaches, and restlessness. One easy way to activate this point is by massaging it firmly in a circular motion with the first and middle fingers.

# BODY-BASED THERAPIES

Our body is complex yet wonderfully orchestrated. Some of its functions are automated while others are the result of our conscious needs, desires, wishes, or reactions. We often think we are in full control of our body's functions and to a certain degree, we are. That is if we can take control of our brain and our mind by monitoring and measuring what is going on inside our bodies. Biofeedback and neurofeedback can help us capture and use the information given by our body to take control and achieve better sleep.

## BIOFEEDBACK THERAPIES

Biofeedback therapy is a technique designed to give patients control over their own body, by letting them observe, understand, and take control of the physiological signs related to their stress and other health issues. Monitoring is done using non-invasive electronic devices and sensors, which take measurements then feed back individual bio-data. This helps raise self-awareness until an individual learns to take voluntary mind control of some of their biological and physiological functions, which has been proven to treat certain medical or psychological conditions, including insomnia. The learning process takes some time over a series of sessions either at a physical therapy facility, a medical center, or hospital.

### MEASUREMENT RESPONSE AND LEARNING

Biofeedback collects and shows the data related to your stress levels, then it is up to you to connect your brain's understanding with the necessary steps to calm down and relax both physically and mentally. Here are the functions that can be measured with biofeedback sensors:

+ Breathing
+ Heart rate
+ Heart rate variability
+ Skin temperature
+ Body temperature

+ Sweating
+ Blood pressure
+ Muscle tension
+ Brain waves
+ Sleep stages

Measuring these physical signals and physiological processes provides important evidence of your stress and anxiety levels, the intensity of your emotions, the quality and duration of your sleep, your state of muscular tension, and whether you are relaxed or not. Static, mobile, and wearable electronic devices can give you this information reliably by displaying your responses captured by sensors positioned on various parts of the body (finger, ear, head, chest, abdomen etc). Wearable devices are portable and simplified measurement tools with an app facilitating biofeedback in the comfort of your own home.

Measurement with home wearable equipment is more limited and perhaps not entirely accurate, but the principle is the same: Data appears on an electronic display or computer monitor, or is communicated as sound feedback, which will help establish a mind-body connection and train you to master your own body. You can then take action to relax, stay calm, cope, or practice self-care until these uncomfortable signs disappear, whether during the day, before going to bed, or in the middle of the night.

An elevated and irregular heart rate, sweaty palms, and shallow breathing for example, indicate physiological stress and anxiety. Rapid brain waves while in bed preparing for sleep can indicate an agitated, overstimulated, and overactive mind—perhaps you are ruminating on a stressful situation at work, trying to solve a problem, worrying about paying the bills, or mentally compiling a to-do list for the next day.

Tracking such responses alone won't resolve the issue, but establishing a mind–body connection can help you be more self-aware and learn how to be serene or control undesirable effects over time, so as to better manage your mental and physical health. For example, you can train to relax the muscles of your neck, shoulder, and back to get rid of spasms or tension. You can learn to ease negative thoughts, anxiety, and stress by visualizing how deep abdominal breathing reduces the physiological stress response.

### NEUROFEEDBACK: THE BRAIN
Neurofeedback is a type of biofeedback that monitors specific brain waves and the central nervous system with sensors or electrodes placed on the head or scalp. With training, a patient can modify their physical response and regulate their brain activity based on the data fed back through the measurement instruments. Some devices can also emit relaxing or sleep-inducing sounds in real time in response to overactive brain waves.

By becoming aware of the impact a movement, thought, or feeling can have on your brain waves, it is possible to increase your coping and adaptation skills, and facilitate your sleep. The sensors and electrodes on your scalp or head measure brain wave frequencies and let you know when your brain is active as opposed to relaxed. Some EEG (an electroencephalogram that evaluates electrical activity in the brain) neurofeedback headbands or headsets can produce sounds letting you know when your brain waves are slowing down, indicating that your mind is calm and ready for sleep. Some of the sounds emitted are often designed to send you into an even deeper sleep (see page 181).

## PNEUMOGRAPHIC BIOFEEDBACK: THE BREATH

Steadily slowing down your breathing pattern, particularly with deep abdominal breathing, is one of the most efficient relaxation and sleep techniques (see pages 76-77). It is used to calm panic attacks and help you fall asleep faster. Pneumographic biofeedback measures abdominal versus chest breathing, which can help train a patient to improve their ability to relax and calm their nervous system. The breath is measured with a companion app, which can respond to an active mind in real time with guided breathing instructions.

## HEART RATE VARIABILITY (HRV) BIOFEEDBACK: THE HEART

One of the physiological responses seen during sleep onset (when you fall asleep) is the slowing down of the heart rate. On waking up, or if there is a need to become active, exercise, run away from danger, or deal with a stressful situation, the heart rate increases. Both are natural and healthy cardiovascular and physiological responses. A healthy heart rate should be variable, showing our capacity to adapt and be responsive to situations.

The oscillations in heart rate are partly driven by our breathing; the heart rate tends to increase when inhaling, and decrease when exhaling, at about mid-breath in both cases. Heart rate variability (HRV) biofeedback brings harmony between the heart rate and the breath, and trains us to activate the parasympathetic nervous system (see page 22), which leads to relaxation. This feedback technique measuring acute changes, or lack thereof, has been used to help conditions linked to physiological systems, such as pain and blood pressure control, as well as psychological conditions such as anxiety, chronic stress, panic attacks, post-traumatic stress disorder (PTSD), and depression, all of which are major sleep disrupters.

## COMBINING BIOFEEDBACK WITH RELAXATION TECHNIQUES

Consider combining practical body-mind relaxation techniques described in this book to enhance the results from biofeedback training. This will go a long way to helping you progress and take more mind control over your body and your psyche to be able to fall asleep.

For example combine with:

+ Breathwork (see pages 76-77)
+ Body scanning (see page 79)
+ Progressive muscle relaxation (see pages 78-79)
+ Visualization (see page 81)
+ Mind-control practices (see pages 90-92)
+ Psycho-emotional healing therapies (see pages 92-94)

# WATER-BASED THERAPIES

For most of us, water has a positive and healing effect whether we see it, feel it on our skin, bathe in it, drink it, or hear it. Water naturally makes us feel calmer and gives us a sense of tranquility. Is it linked to our first conscious experience as a fetus floating in the womb? Or is it perhaps related to the fact that on average over 50 percent (the range is 40 to 70 percent depending on our age and gender) of our body composition is made of water? Is it the soothing sensory experience water gives us when it touches our bodies externally or internally? Or does our brain subconsciously just know that water is good for us?

## HYDROTHERAPY

What natural health practitioners, holistic therapists, and some scientists alike have discovered is that water also has healing properties and can help prevent illnesses. It is always recommended to first consult your physician or trained practitioner before proceeding with hydrotherapy.

*Hydro* comes from an ancient Greek word for water. In fact, therapeutic treatments using water are as ancient as mankind, and part of medicinal systems in many ancient and current cultures around the world as a complementary or alternative medicine to treat various ailments. Hydrotherapy is the use of water either externally or internally in any form—warm, hot, cold, or iced—to improve health and well-being. It is prescribed individually with different durations, pressure levels, body location, and frequency.

A scientific review of clinical studies and literature concluded that hydrotherapy is widely used to treat a large range of ailments and, even though there is a lack of understanding of how this works, it confirmed that these healing effects are scientifically evidence-based[8].

## THERMAL CURES

These consist of bathing in hot or cold-water springs, just as ancient Greeks and Romans regularly did, not only to cleanse but also to cure various musculoskeletal ailments, rheumatism and skin diseases, stimulate blood circulation and digestion, and facilitate relaxation. Most patients report much better sleep as an additional benefit of such treatments.

## AQUATIC OR POOL THERAPY

This takes place in a pool or other aquatic setting and is mostly prescribed to support physical rehabilitation, but it is well known for reducing stress and promoting relaxation. This requires supervision from a medically and therapeutically trained professional and is not to be confused with aquatic exercise or aqua gym.

## BALNEOTHERAPY

This consists of immersing patients in waters containing minerals or covering them in wet mud, which is rich in minerals. Soaking in hot or cold mineral-rich pools is used to reduce pain, regulate hormonal fluctuations, facilitate digestion, and stimulate other physiological processes. It also contributes to improving sleep.

## HYDROMASSAGE THERAPY

This treatment consists of applying a high-pressure stream of water as a massage, which is typically warmer and much more powerful than in a whirlpool or jacuzzi. It reduces stress and muscular tension, while inducing relaxation and good-quality sleep. Warm water will trigger the body's temperature to increase

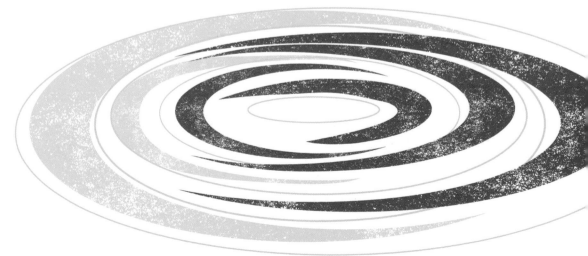

then decrease, which the brain perceives as one of the signals indicating it is time to go to sleep. Such treatment also helps lower the levels of the stress hormone cortisol, relieve physical pain, and improve blood circulation.

## WARM OR HOT BATHS

Soaking in warm or hot water about 90 to 120 minutes before bedtime is an efficient way to fall asleep faster and deeper. The body's internal temperature increases as a result, and it then takes a couple of hours for it to drop gradually. This physiological process makes us feel drowsy and sleepy faster. A healthy bath temperature is generally about 100°F and in any case should not be higher than 104°F. It is important to allow enough time for the body to cool down, since overheating while in bed will prevent sleep. It is also essential to drink water to avoid dehydration, but to do so well before bedtime to avoid bathroom trips during the night. Hot tubs help lower blood pressure, slow down heart rate, relax body tension, soothe painful joints, and stimulate the release of endorphins, all of which result in more restful sleep.

## THALASSOTHERAPY

Thalassotherapy comes from the Greek word *thalassa*, which means "sea," and is the therapeutic use of seawater for cosmetic and health treatments. The healing benefits of seawater have been celebrated since ancient times, whether to disinfect wounds or provide pain relief.

Thalassotherapy is hydrotherapy with seawater combined with the healing properties of other elements such as algae, seaweed, marine mud, beach, coastal air, and marine climate. It is believed that trace elements and minerals can penetrate through the skin's open pores, which help restore chemical balance in the body.

A study investigated the effects of thalassotherapy on healthy workers by giving them 3 days of a wide range of thalassotherapy treatments combined with sleep management. This resulted in immediate beneficial effects on sleep duration, mood, anxiety, fatigue, general well-being, and daytime sleepiness. Positive effects were still observed up to 3 days post treatment.[9]

## FLOATING THERAPY

Floating on tranquil water is so calming that it is said to slow down brain waves, lower biochemicals related to stress and anxiety, and release painkiller endorphins. Whether floating in a bathtub, lake, swimming pool, or in the sea, this provides a moment of peace, quietness, and weightless bliss. Another option is to use floating therapy tanks, where you can spend an hour in an enclosed booth filled with salted water in either full darkness or dimmed lighting. This moment of self-care and time alone has proven to be restful and restorative and to help support quality sleep.

# ENERGY-HEALING THERAPIES

The principle behind energy-based therapies is to heal a patient using "vital energy," which proponents believe flows within and around the body. Despite the lack of support from Western scientists, and even though it has been practiced for thousands of years in Asian, Indian, and African cultures, this approach is becoming more popular in Western culture. The objective is to restore our natural energetic balance and mind–body well-being to treat medical conditions and psychological disturbances, while reducing stress and anxiety.

## REFLEXOLOGY

Reflexology has origins in traditional Chinese medicine (see pages 128-134) and is reminiscent of acupressure, as it uses pressure on specific points on the body to promote healing and relaxation with a focus on the hands, feet, face, and ears. The idea is that these body parts act as a map to the rest of the body, with certain points connected to organs, glands, and tissues via the nervous system. Reflexology points are stimulated with a specialized and focused light-pressure massage repeated in several sessions over a few weeks, and this is thought to be an effective treatment to help with sleep.

## REIKI

Reiki is originally a Japanese method that follows similar energetic principles to those of Ayurveda and traditional Chinese medicine. In this complementary or alternative energy-healing therapy, the practitioner hovers their hands over various parts of the body to tune into its natural energy fields and channels—an energy transfer takes place, which often creates a sensation of warmth. Occasionally the therapist may apply very light pressure as well. During the therapy, the patient lies fully clothed on a massage table or sits comfortably. This technique helps restore the flow of energy, in a similar way to acupuncture, acupressure, and marma therapy. It promotes the natural ability to heal and is said to relieve physical or psychological imbalances and illnesses, often resulting in people feeling more relaxed and less stressed.

## "TOUCH" THERAPIES

With healing touch therapy, a trained healer places and moves their hands over different parts of the body, but without actually touching the patient, to treat a wide range of medical and mental health conditions. In therapeutic touch therapy, another energy-healing technique, the practitioner uses gentle touch to heal. Both therapies are said to reduce anxiety and contribute to the recovery from certain conditions, although there is little support from the scientific community to confirm this. Some pilot studies have shown good results in patients with chronic stress and anxiety, although they were criticized for not having observed the best methodology and it's unclear whether the positive results were due to a placebo effect or not.

## ENERGETIC CORD-CUTTING

Sometimes, the reason why we are unable to sleep at night is because of unhealthy relationships we hang on to, which no longer serve us. Doing so drains our energy or focuses it on the wrong things or people. Holding onto it can create obsessive behavior and thinking patterns, which stay with us through the night and can prevent us from sleeping soundly. An energetic cord-cutting ceremony is said to help with letting go and releasing the ties with anything or anyone holding you back or having a negative impact on you. This spiritual ritual can be done alone or with the help of an energy healer. Simply explained, it involves visualizing the energetic cord that connects and binds you to the person you would like to let go of and imagine cutting it with a sharp object or burning it with a candle. This can be repeated several times until a feeling of lightness and freedom arises, which could be the key to a good night's sleep.

## CRYSTAL HEALING THERAPY

Certain crystals, gems, and healing stones are said to have powerful healing properties and connect us with the earth's grounding energy. They are meant to transmit their properties to us energetically speaking and help restore balance and health. Different stones and crystals have different effects, but all aim to resolve and heal physical, emotional, and spiritual issues. It is recommended to keep them close by carrying them or wearing them as necklaces or bracelets, or by placing them in the bedroom. Healers exercise words of caution, however, saying that a crystal's powerful energy can keep us awake at night, in which case it should be placed further away from the bed or replaced with a smaller stone. Here are a few of the crystals and stones recommended to help improve sleep:

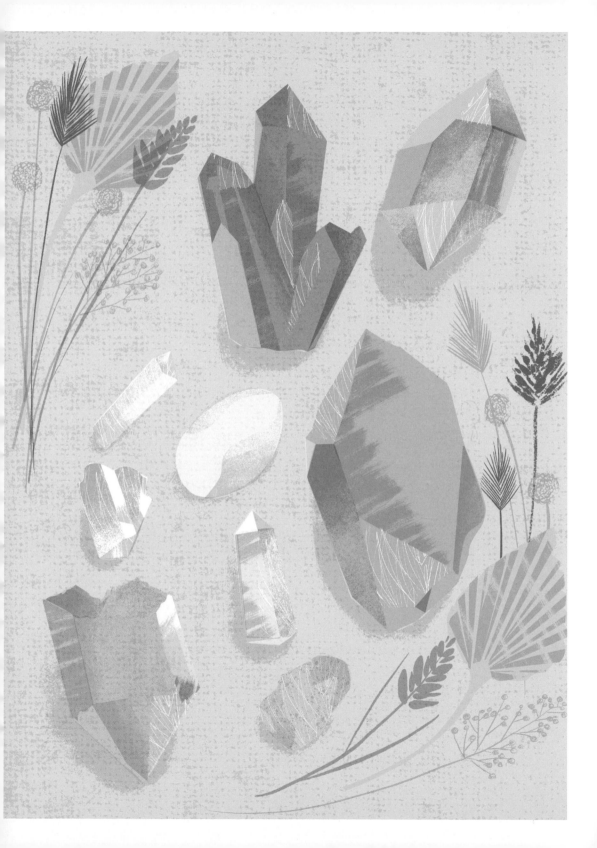

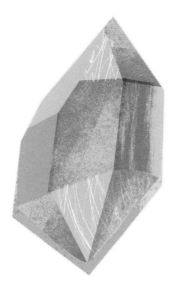

+ **AMETHYST**: A gorgeous purple quartz that promotes sleep by diffusing stress and negative emotions and providing protection.
+ **CELESTITE**: A beautiful blue crystal that brings calm, inner peace, harmony, and serenity. It is also uplifting.
+ **LEPIDOLITE**: An intriguing purplish-pink or lilac crystal that balances the mind, relieves stressful emotions, and brings peace.

## CONTACT-BASED THERAPIES

Human touch is essential to our mental and physical health and development. Starting in childhood, babies who lack contact and emotional engagement have much higher levels of the stress hormone cortisol and lower levels of oxytocin and vasopressin (hormones linked to emotional and social bonding). Skin-to-skin contact calms babies and helps them sleep better.

According to the Touch Research Institute at the University of Miami School of Medicine, tactile interactions generate a positive physiological response necessary to our well-being. Moving the skin stimulates skin sensors, which send signals to the vagus nerve responsible for switching on our parasympathetic nervous system (see page 22), leading to a state of relaxation essential for sleep. A survey conducted by the institute during the 2020 coronavirus lockdown showed that 42 percent of people surveyed felt deprived of touch, and 97 percent of the sample experienced sleep disturbances.[10]

Touch given to a consenting individual is good physiologically: It calms down the nervous system, lowers the levels of stress hormones, slows down heart rate and blood pressure, increases the release of serotonin and oxytocin (respectively, the happy and love hormones). In other words, moving the skin before bedtime is conducive to an excellent night's sleep.

### MASSAGE THERAPY

Massage therapy has been practiced around the world for thousands of years for a wide range of reasons: to reduce stress, relieve muscular tension and pain, increase mobility and flexibility, improve blood circulation, relax mind and body, heal, cure, and rejuvenate. A massage is a hands-on technique applying pressure on and manipulating the skin, muscles, and soft tissues of the entire body. The practitioner uses very specific techniques to rub, manipulate, and stretch body parts in turn, from scalp to toes. There are many massage techniques, methods, approaches, and often massage therapists combine two or more to provide the best treatment—for example, acupressure (see pages 134–135), marma points therapy (see pages 122–124), and reflexology (see page 141). There is also the option to self-massage, wherever practical, which can be done while in bed just before falling asleep. Massaging the scalp, neck, shoulders, back, forearms, hands, and feet is good for sleep, as we tend to hold the most tension around these important healing points, which promote sleep when activated.

## CRANIOSACRAL THERAPY

Craniosacral therapy is a relatively recent therapy that consists of applying very gentle hands-on pressure to the skull, spine, and pelvis to facilitate the flow and circulation of cerebrospinal fluid—the fluid that surrounds and cushions the brain and spinal cord. Such light touch manipulations are meant to support the entire body's healing and provide profound health benefits including stress management, central nervous system support, and chronic fatigue

relief. Craniosacral therapy is generally performed by osteopaths, chiropractors, and massage therapists.

## CUDDLE THERAPY

Hugging and cuddling are generally synonymous with feeling good and with happy moments in our lives, yet it seems that modern life does not provide enough opportunities to create physical human connections, even though we are digitally hyperconnected with others. Do you remember the last time you held your partner or a close friend for a prolonged time? Have you ever held a stranger to console them or celebrate something joyful? Has hugging or cuddling someone become too awkward or risky because of possible misinterpretation?

Our basic human need for safe physical contact has given way to a new wave of therapy called cuddle therapy provided by professional cuddlers. The benefit of platonic and innocent touch is to create an actual connection and share a moment together with another person while being in the present moment. Cuddle therapy releases oxytocin, the hormone related to love, social bonding, and sexual activity. There is evidence that this "cuddle" hormone influences sleep processes and that, combined with a sense of safety, it helps release body tension and regulates the breath and heart rate by creating a sense of calm, all of which is conducive to good sleep.

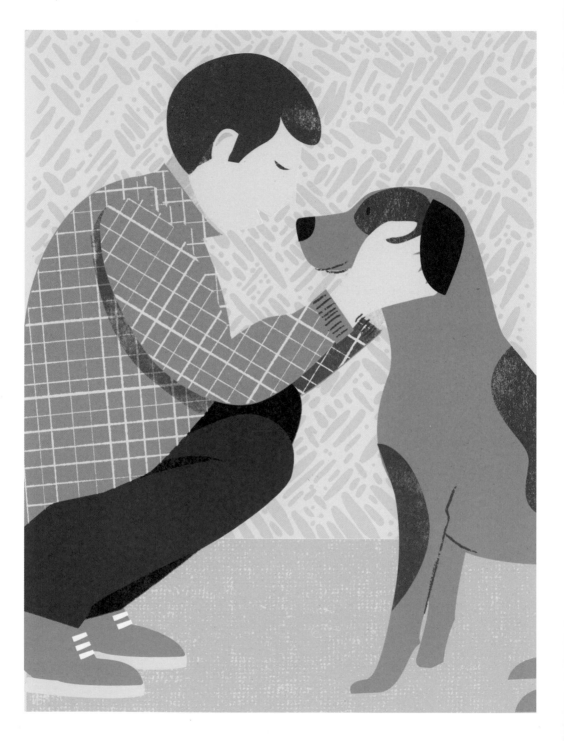

Cuddle sessions consist of connecting with a therapist or someone else in a therapy group. Sessions proceed in several stages to give participants the time to adjust to such unfamiliar yet harmless non-sexual intimacy: Getting to know each other's background, obtaining consent before holding hands, eyes closed, then standing and embracing someone, or laying down in a spooning position until the tension and awkwardness pass.

## ANIMAL-ASSISTED THERAPY

Sharing our lives with a pet is excellent for companionship and nurturing needs. Therapy dogs, for example, can be "prescribed" to give emotional support, distraction, and stimulation to distressed, depressed, elderly, or lonely people. Animal-assisted therapy (AAT) has been shown to improve general health and well-being and can help those with special needs by giving them a sense of calm and focus. In addition to the incredible and supportive relationship we can build with our furry or feathery friends, petting an animal can create pressure stimulation on the skin and promote the release of oxytocin as a physiological reaction leading to a very relaxed state. For some of us, it also provides a sense of safety, which is essential to fall asleep, as long as your pet doesn't disrupt your sleep during the night (see page 62).

## SHARING YOUR BED

Ending this section on contact-based therapies without reflecting on the benefits of sleeping together would not do it justice! Sharing your bed with someone has many benefits. It:

+ Allows you to shift your mental focus to you both as a couple, rather than being trapped in your own obsessive thoughts.
+ Creates a sense of well-being by releasing oxytocin, the cuddle and love hormone.
+ Makes you feel safe, which contributes to lowering the stress hormone cortisol, an essential factor to fall asleep.
+ Keeps you warm in winter while in bed, how nice . . .

This is a wonderful combination of benefits, which can lead to a brilliant night's sleep. However, if sharing your bed doesn't work for you, turn to pages 61–63 for some possible solutions.

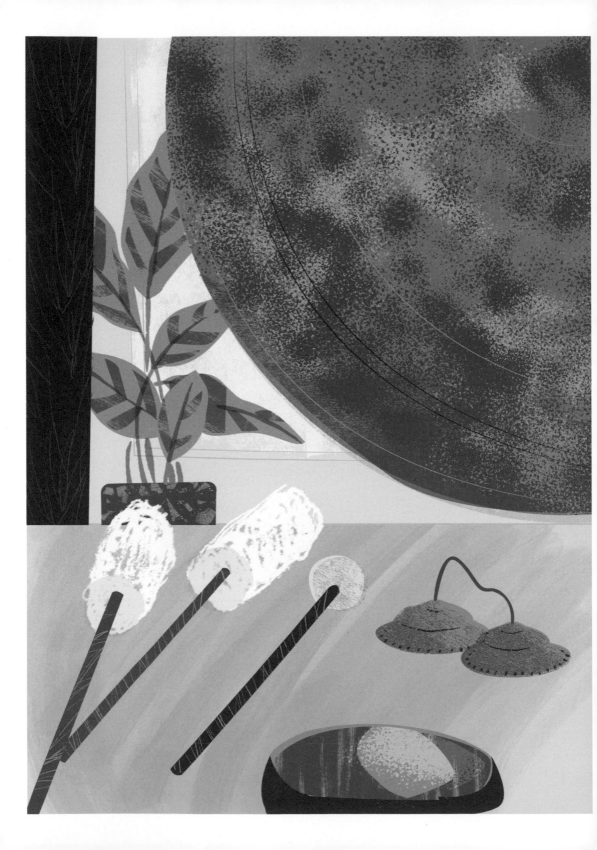

# SOUND ASLEEP

Research shows that sound waves can affect brain-wave activity, and the slower and lower the frequency of the brain waves, the deeper our state of relaxation and sleep becomes. The process of tuning the brain with sounds is called brain entrainment, which means that when exposed to sound waves at certain frequencies, brain-wave patterns adjust to synchronize with them. Sound therapy uses frequencies, sounds, music, and instruments combined with breathing and introspective techniques to improve our general well-being. By affecting our psychology, neurology, and physiology, sound therapy can help us manage our energy levels, mental health, physical health, and our ability to calm down. The ideas in this section will show how sound therapy can help you achieve longer, better, and more restorative sleep.

## FAMILIAR AND COMFORTING SOUNDS

Our brain continues to register and process sounds at a basic level even when we are asleep. This is most probably an evolutionary ability so that our ancestors could be aware of any looming predators and quickly wake up to defend themselves. While we sleep, the brain filters many sounds and decides what is worth waking up for and, over time, it learns to recognize sounds that are either unusual, relevant, require attention, or are emotionally charged. These will systematically wake us up and disrupt our sleep.

We become more sensitive to unexpected sounds in the light sleep stages than when we are in deep sleep— and even more so in the second half of the night, when light sleep cycles are longer. The level to which we are affected depends on how we feel about the sounds we hear while we are unconscious.

From a young age, children fall asleep when hearing the comforting sounds they have grown accustomed to, such as their mother singing a lullaby or their father reading a bedtime story. Take a moment to reflect and remember your favorite bedtime sounds or any pleasant sounds that made you feel safe, serene, comforted, and relaxed. For some the sound of rain will contribute to better sleep, for others it might be the noisy sound of traffic or a plane. It all depends on what you are used to and what your mental association is with that sound. As adults we should pay attention to and nurture the only sense that stays "awake" while we sleep.

# HEALING SOUNDS

The healing power of therapeutic tones, vibrations, frequencies, and soundscapes, also known as psychoacoustics and neuroacoustics, affect our brain waves and our mood and can help improve our sleep. We hear them, but we also feel them as vibrations throughout our body. These sounds can bring physical and emotional balance, joy, happiness, energy, peace, safety, relaxation, comfort, and a space for healing. Listening to them is particularly efficient when combined with breathwork (see pages 76-79). That said, each of us might react differently to various auditory techniques.

You can find the suggestions in this section on a wide number of digital apps, free and paid for streaming services, and websites distributing recordings of meditation, music, video, and sound recordings—or in a CD or DVD format if that is more practical for you. Experiment with a variety of sounds until you discover the ones you find most relaxing and reassuring. Identify the ones that facilitate the onset of sleep or relax you back into sleep in the middle of the night. Select a comfortable volume, preferably low, so as not to prevent you from entering deep sleep. If you are worried about disturbing your partner or others living with you, use comfortable headphones for sleep or pillow speakers (see the Sleep Tech information on pages 177-187).

To protect your hearing, medical advice is as follows:

+ Use noise-canceling earphones or headphones rather than turning the volume up to block out outside noise.
+ Turn the volume up just enough so you can hear comfortably, but no higher—sounds below 70 dB are generally considered safe, but opt for much lower volume (30 dB or less).
+ Don't listen to music or sounds at more than 60 percent of the maximum volume (see below)—some devices have settings you can use to limit the volume automatically.
+ Avoid using earphones or headphones for more than an hour at a time—take a break for at least 5 minutes every hour.

Volume range in decibels (dB):
+ Whispering: 30 dB
+ Conversation: 60 dB
+ Busy traffic: 70-85 dB
+ Motorbike: 90 dB
+ Listening to music on full volume through headphones: 100-110 dB
+ Plane taking off: 120 dB

# NEUROACOUSTICS

Neuroacoustics was most likely invented by Dr. Jeffrey Thompson, a leading sound healing researcher, who has been exploring the therapeutic application of sound for decades. His research is well known for demonstrating the use of healing sounds as a means to impact brain waves and the autonomous nervous system, and neuroacoustics has become a complementary therapy for certain medical and mental illnesses such as cardiovascular diseases, cancer, stress, and depression.

Noises you are very familiar with and used to hearing, that don't bother you during the day, can become a nuisance when you hear them while you're in bed and everything else is quiet. Think of a door slamming, a radiator clicking, a leaky faucet drip-dropping water. A number of musicians and audio engineers combined forces with neuroscientists to record some helpful sonic solutions that can help you sleep by masking environmental noises or by impacting your brain positively toward better sleep. Here are a few examples:

## WHITE NOISE

White noise minimizes the difference between background sounds and an unexpected abrupt sound, so that the sudden noise is masked and doesn't disrupt your sleep. It is a mix of all audible frequencies and a constant ambient sound. Environmental sounds such as waterfalls, rivers flowing, fountains, rainfall, and ocean waves are some of the best examples of natural white noise. Sound conditioners or white noise machines are often used to create ongoing and consistent simulated background sounds throughout the night. However, any other device producing a similar steady environmental sound, such as humidifiers, dehumidifiers, electrical fans, air purifiers, and air conditioners can also create the effect of covering up outdoor and indoor noise. The same goes for the steady humming noise of machinery, cars, planes, or drones. Experiment and select the noise that works best for you, and ensure it is neither too quiet nor too loud. White noise is also often used to treat a medical condition called tinnitus (perception of noise or ringing in your ears), which can disturb sleep when everything around us is quiet at night.

Many people fall asleep with the television on, treating it as a white noise, but it isn't—the sounds from TV and films are unpredictable and can vary drastically in terms of volume, types, and regularity. They are much more likely

---

CAUTION: Hearing loss due to aging is unavoidable, but hearing loss due to exposure to loud noises can be avoided.

Pregnant women and anyone with mental health or neurologic disorders are advised not to undertake sound therapy without consulting a medical healthcare professional. In general, always exercise caution and consult a doctor for further advice.

to wake you up at some point, even if it is just to switch the TV off. If you find that you are sleeping fine throughout the night and feel totally refreshed the next day, then you can probably continue sleeping with the TV on, although it is not advisable. If you don't sleep well, then the general recommendation is not to have a TV in your bedroom and certainly not to leave it on as you fall asleep.

## PINK NOISE

Pink noise is similar to white noise, but it is a deeper sound, with more bass. They differ because white noise has an equal power per hertz throughout all frequencies (a mix of all audible frequencies), while for pink noise, the power per hertz density decreases as the frequency increases. Pink noise slows down and regulates the brain waves making it easier to fall asleep. Pink noise is often found in nature, such as ocean waves crashing on the beach, a steady rain falling on the pavement, or wind blowing through tree leaves. Scientific studies[1] have shown that pink noise increases slow-wave activity linked to deep sleep and dramatically improves memory in healthy older adults, in particular. However, both white noise and pink noise help—it's really a matter of individual preference and response, so try them both and see which one is most effective for you.

## BINAURAL BEATS

Binaural beats are a combination of sound frequencies, which are reported to be soothing, relaxing, and even conducive to falling asleep for many. Such audio recordings, when played through headphones, stimulate the right and left ear simultaneously with two different but almost equivalent pure tones, with slightly different frequencies to create the perception of a single new frequency tone. The sounds themselves are not the most pleasant to listen to, but seem to be highly effective for some people and are worth a try. The brain responses to binaural beats remain controversial, but they have been studied and proven to be effective at slowing down and synchronizing brain waves, inducing a relaxed and meditative state within a short duration.[2] It is thought that this type of sonic activation alternates evenly and rhythmically between the left and right sides of the brain, causing them to resonate and synchronize.

## BRAIN HEMISPHERE SYNCHRONIZATION (BHS)

This works by slowly panning a sound from one ear to the other back and forth to synchronize the brain waves of each brain hemisphere. The left hemisphere is the verbal, analytical and thinking side, and the right hemisphere is the creative, visual, intuitive, and emotional side.

In theory, by building an auditory bridge between the right and left hemispheres of your brain, such sound creates a sense of coordination, balance, relaxation, and helps you wind down and therefore sleep better.

# PSYCHOACOUSTICS

Psychoacoustics is the scientific study of sound perception—more specifically, the science of studying the physical and psychological human interpretations and responses associated with sound (including noise, speech, and music). In this section, we will focus on the psychological impact of sound when it comes to improving our sleep.

## AUTONOMOUS SENSORY MERIDIAN RESPONSE (ASMR)

According to its followers, ASMR can reduce insomnia, panic attacks, stress, and anxiety and generate intense euphoria. It was born out of an online community sharing experiences on these sensations and has become a YouTube phenomenon with millions of viewers. ASMR is often referred to as a "mental massage" or a "head orgasm." The sounds are reported to trigger soothing tingling physical and/or psychological sensations, making the listener feel deeply relaxed enough to nod off and fall asleep. Apparently, there are specific stimuli that give pleasurable sensations to the listener or viewer. ASMR video and audio recordings are widely available on YouTube, relaxation apps, and as podcasts.

The experience includes gentle yet audible sounds, voices, and demonstrations of familiar situations. Examples of the sounds are breathy whispers, a moist tongue against the palate, lips popping or smacking, fluttering sounds, rubbing on a surface, skin, or object, tapping or clicking noises, towel-folding, chewing crunchy or wet foods, scratching surfaces, brushing hair, painting a canvas, and so on. In visual ASMR, the presenters appear to be totally focused on you and the sensations they can generate in you, sometimes even performing a role-play and generally making slow and repetitive movements alongside their sounds. The sessions often last about 30 minutes and should be listened to with headphones for an immersive experience.

This technique may not work for everyone, but the scientific theory behind ASMR is that the sounds trigger the release of oxytocin, endorphins, dopamine, and serotonin, promoting feelings of love, bonding, relaxation, euphoria, bliss, and well-being. The physical sensations are described by ASMR University as "light and pleasurable tingles, sparkles, fuzziness, or waves of relaxation in the head, neck, spine, and throughout the rest of the body" and the psychological sensations as "deep and soothing feelings of relaxation, calmness, comfort, peacefulness, restfulness, or sleepiness."

## GUIDED AUDIO RECORDINGS

Listening to spoken words, guided instructions, or fictional stories is an effective way to fall asleep for many people. The human voice has proven to be an efficient auditory tool helping those unable to sleep well. The messages delivered need to be gentle and not overly intellectually stimulating, provocative, or exciting. Again, it is best to try different options and decide for yourself what works best for you.

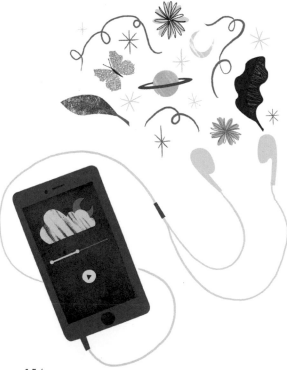

### BEDTIME STORIES FOR ADULTS OR CHILDREN

Reading stories to children is a common bedtime ritual that has recently become more popular with adults. Meditation apps and websites have introduced sleep storytelling to help adults relax at bedtime. In fact, there are now specialized sleep writers whose evening stories are often read out by celebrities and heard by millions of listeners on an ongoing basis. The stories are written in such a way that the listener is not likely to stay awake until the end of the story. Imagery and sensorial descriptions are at the core of the writing technique. The objective is to lead the listeners to visualize and imagine the story and engage all of their senses, with a sense of comfort, relaxation, and pleasure without overly stimulating them. The reason why this works for many adults might also be because it reminds them of comforting childhood moments with their parents by their side, or because the human voice provides a social presence needed for a sense of safety and protection.

### PODCASTS

The podcast industry discovered that listeners used certain podcasts as a means to fall asleep. Whether fictional tales, factual documentaries, or descriptive narratives, it appears that podcasts can either engage, inform, or relax their followers depending on the level of stimulation they experience. In a way, these aren't dissimilar to bedtime stories since they help cover surrounding noises, provide a sense of calm, and give the illusion of a comforting presence by your bedside.

### GUIDED RELAXATION RECORDINGS

The following techniques are described in the Beditation section (see pages 75-85) as some of the most effective ways to fall asleep. Guiding yourself through these techniques can require a mental effort if you are not used to them, so passively listening to someone else's voice instructing you on what you need to do, can in itself, make you relax and take away some of the strain. Recordings of these techniques are widely available. They usually last from 10 minutes to an hour, and often combine all the techniques. They are occasionally supplemented with background sounds or music.

+ Guided progressive muscle relaxation (PMR): A technique of contracting and releasing muscles, while breathing sequentially (see pages 78-79).
+ Guided meditation: A practice of focusing your mind in silence, especially for spiritual reasons or mind management in order to achieve clarity and calm (see pages 90-92).
+ Guided imagery: A relaxation method focusing the mind on visual and sensorial descriptions and sensations (see pages 90-92).

## OTHER POPULAR SOUNDSCAPES FOR SLEEP

### NATURE SOUND RECORDINGS

Mother Nature has so much to offer and her sounds give us many signals that our brains can perceive as good or bad, comforting or scary. Generally the following nature sounds evoke a peaceful and comforting experience: ocean waves crashing on a beach, a spring river streaming down a mountain, large river birds tweeting, rocky waterfalls, heavy tropical rain, light drizzle rain, heavy coastal wind, light desert breeze, afternoon forest atmosphere, outdoor camping or beach bonfires, thunderstorms, underwater ocean sounds, evening crickets chirping, and owls hooting.

### EVERYDAY SOUND RECORDINGS

Some of us would rather hear the sounds of a familiar everyday environment, such as highway traffic, trains, washing machines, fire crackling in fireplaces, boats in harbors, windy rain tapping at our windows, airplanes taking off.

### WIND CHIMES

The sound of wind chimes can create a peaceful auditory background conducive to relaxation and sleep. They were traditionally hung to chase away evil spirits and today are commonly used to help the flow of energy in homes.

## SOUND BATHS

A sound bath is an ancient yet unique and fully immersive healing experience. It is as unique as the sound therapist who orchestrates it on the day. Each session is "performed" and improvised live for an audience whose members are generally lying down on mats or comfortable mattresses to receive this vibrant and sonic experience. Sometimes eye pillows or eye masks and blankets are given to participants to make them comfortable and fully introspective.

During an hour-long session the sound therapist produces many sounds and vibrations in succession, increasing and decreasing their volume and intensity throughout. These sounds are intense and powerful, yet can be very relaxing and healing. Some listeners may even fall asleep during the session, despite the loudness of the experience. Sound baths generally slow down our brain waves and may bring up some emotions in the process. The vibrations and frequencies of sound baths penetrate our bodies and our brains through the conduit of our ears and our flesh, but some believe they also touch our souls.

Sound baths simplify and focus our thoughts, as the sound is louder than our thoughts. It is believed that they also help align and tune our own energetic vibrations with the universe. Besides their calming effect, sound baths may reduce stress, anxiety, and emotional imbalance, while clearing the subconscious mind from negative thoughts and energies.

The therapist may use one of or a combination of the following instruments and objects:

+ Tuning forks
+ Gongs
+ Crystal singing bowls
+ Tibetan bowls
+ Chimes
+ Shruti box
+ Drums
+ Bells

## MUSIC AS SLEEP THERAPY

Scientific researchers found evidence to support that music improves sleep quality for chronic insomnia sufferers[3]. Listening to soothing and soft music helps reduce anxiety, depression, and improves our mood. It seems to have an effect on the parasympathetic nervous system (see page 22) and triggers our muscles to relax. Music is used as a complementary therapy to Western medicine for a multitude of medical conditions such as cancer, dementia, and pain. It can slow breathing, lower blood pressure, calm the nervous system, and even lower your heart rate and can also increase feel-good hormones serotonin and oxytocin or decrease stress hormone cortisol.

For babies and children, popular lullabies are part of the evening wind-down routine signaling to the brain it's bedtime and safe to fall asleep.

A study[4] conducted by Mattress Advisor collected data on 20,000 sleep and relaxation playlists on Spotify and found that listeners were using Spotify to wind down and fall asleep. Interestingly C was the top musical key appearing in this research.

Specialized sleep music composers have teamed up with neuroscientists to create soundscapes made up of original music mixed with neuroacoustic (see pages 150-153) and psychoacoustic sounds, creating a pleasing and relaxing effect on the brain, making you fall asleep or be in between wakefulness and sleep. Max Richter is perhaps the most popular composer in this genre. His music has no lyrics and is scored for piano, strings, voice, and ambient electronic sounds, with tracks ranging from 10 minutes to 8 hours. Richter describes his popular album *Sleep* as a lullaby for the modern world. He's even offered his music as a live overnight immersive sleep concert. Another notable artist in this genre is Tom Middleton, who has composed psychoacoustic soundscape tracks with a combination of music, noises, and nature sounds, such as ocean and forest sounds designed to engage and relax listeners, until they fall asleep.

Generally, slow, gentle, instrumental music with repetitive patterns and no peaks and lows are best to fall asleep. This is because the brain is responsive to the sounds it hears and tries to align with them. That said, music is a matter of personal choice, therefore decide for yourself the best music for your bedtime sleep routine. The Sleep Foundation suggests looking for music with a rhythm of about 60 to 80 beats per minute (BPM) and preferably instrumental music, without singing or lyrics. It is advisable to avoid music that triggers strong emotions and stressful memories.

## SINGING AND CHANTING

Singing is an interesting pathway toward relaxation and sleep. A lot of us may hum at home, while listening to a song, sing out loud in the shower or at a karaoke bar. Whether we can hold a tune or not, singing feels good. It gives a sense of release and well-being, perhaps because we are expressing emotions and perhaps because singing along makes us feel like we are part of something.

From a biological point of view, though, singing involves abdominal breathing and throat vibrations, especially in low, resonant, and deep notes coming from the lower part of throat. This is a perfect way to trigger the

---

*CAUTION: Listening to loud music through earphones and headphones is one of the biggest dangers to your hearing (see page 150).*

wonderful vagus nerve, the long nerve from the gut to the back of the throat close to the base of the skull. This nerve is critical to our parasympathetic nervous system, the rest and digest state, helping us relax and fall asleep. This nerve is connected to our throat, upper palate, heart, lungs, and parts of our digestive system, and the deeper the singing the easier it is to activate our relaxation system.

While it is of course of a spiritual nature, chanting mantras has a similar physiological effect as singing. The universal "Om" (or "Aum") is perhaps the most popular mantra chanted during meditation or yoga practices. It is quite a deep sound, creating throat vibrations likely to stimulate the relaxing vagus nerve while aligning our intention with our community and the universe. Here are some instructions on how to practice the vibrational "Om" and get the most out of its relaxing effects for better sleep:

1. Sit tall and lengthen the spine, elongating the back of the neck and extending the vagus nerve.
2. Relax and soften the neck and throat to make space for deep vibrations.
3. Bring your awareness to the abdomen and your breathing, using the diaphragm, a respiratory muscle found near the bottom of your rib cage, right below your chest.
4. Inhale and exhale deeply through the nose, feeling the breath massage you internally along the spine and letting the air out humming the "O-m" (or "A-u-m") sound, allowing the throat to vibrate as fully and deeply as possible.

## PLAYING AN INSTRUMENT

Playing an instrument can help relax your mind because when you are learning a new skill, you focus less on your worries. It also sharpens your brain, improving memory and concentration. Studies have found that playing an instrument significantly decreases levels of stress and anxiety, lowering blood pressure and decreasing risk of heart disease and other vascular problems.

Playing certain instruments can help to relieve breathing problems that may affect sleep. Some musical instruments turn out to be effective at toning the respiratory muscles of the upper airways. A study[5] found that musicians who play high-resistance double-reed wind instruments (e.g. oboe, bassoon, and English horn) have a reduced risk of developing OSA (obstructive sleep apnea, snoring and blocked breathing passages preventing deep sleep). Other studies have shown that playing the didgeridoo (a wind instrument from indigenous Australia) helped participants with their apnea after just 4 months of practice.

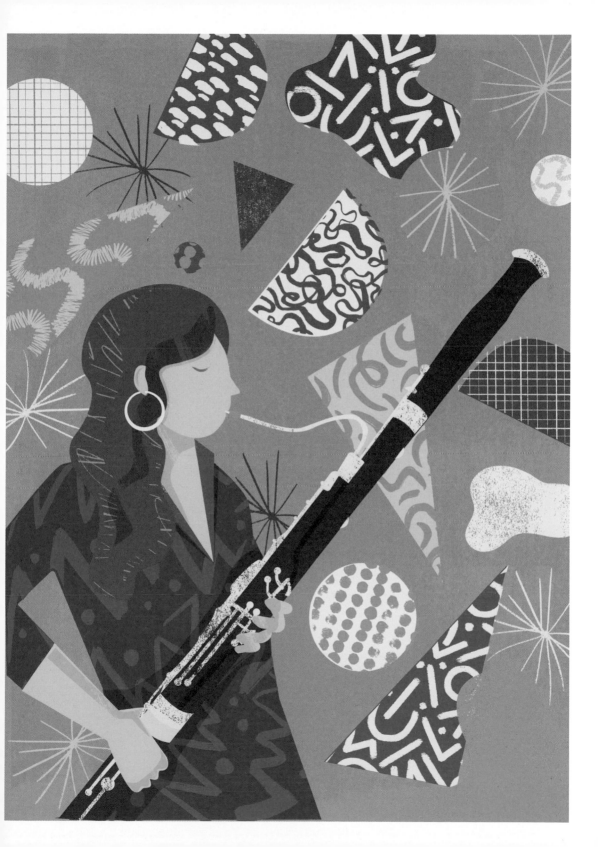

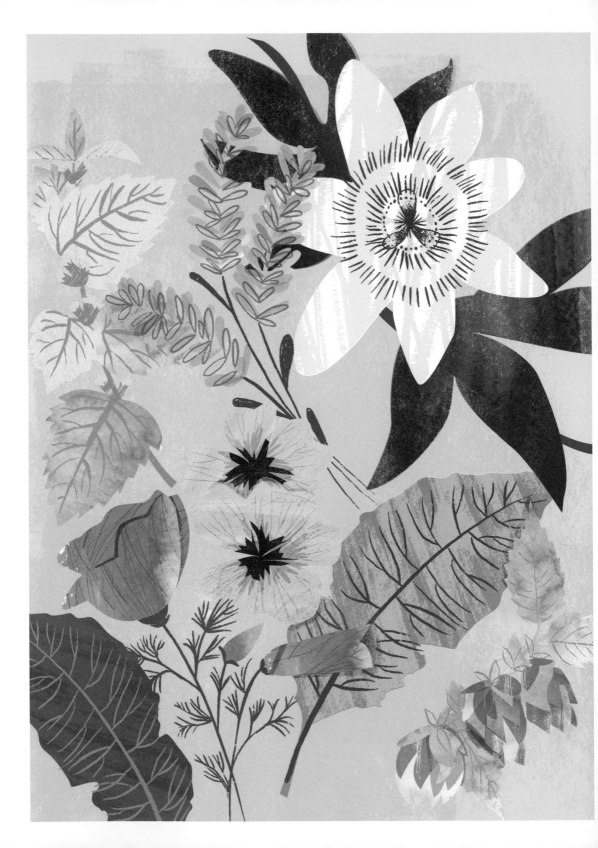

# HEALING PLANTS

The beauty of using herbal remedies is that they support our natural sleep–wake processes. In this section you will find a comprehensive list of wonderful natural medicinal plant herbs that have relaxing, soothing, and sedative properties on the body and the mind and, as a result, will help to improve your sleep. The results usually take longer to obtain than with pharmaceuticals—days and sometimes weeks—but there are minimal side effects. Herbal remedies generally do not cause physical addiction and help gradually to reduce the dependence on pharmaceutical medication for insomnia, but it is important to be aware of the safety guidelines (see overleaf).

## THE USE OF HERBAL REMEDIES

Herbalism uses the knowledge of plants and herbs to help treat diseases and conditions. Plants and herbal remedies have been used to treat all sorts of ailments for centuries. The World Health Organization estimates that 80 percent of people around the world use herbal medicine, but their use is not yet regulated. While there are studies available, there isn't enough scientific evidence for medicinal herbs to be widely accepted by the Western medical profession. However, valerian has been more widely studied in terms of improving the quality of light sleep in particular.[1] Phytotherapy is slightly different as it is a science-based medical practice and thus is distinguished from other approaches that are based on empirical evidence from traditional use.

Herbal remedies are plant-based medicines made from various combinations of plant parts, such as leaves, bark, roots, berries, and flowers, and meant to be suitable for people of any age. Before using herbal remedies, ideally seek the advice of a qualified health professional or therapist who works with medicinal plants, such as a phytotherapist, herbal practitioner, a naturopath doctor, a holistic medical doctor, or an herbal pharmacist. Physicians may also have some knowledge of herbal medicine. If you haven't got access to a professional, herbalism stores can provide leaflets and some guidance.

# SAFETY FIRST

*While herbal remedies are often considered safer than pharmaceuticals, they are potent products with active ingredients, with risks and benefits that need to be assessed and considered.*

+ Exercise caution when using herbal remedies and consult with a trained healthcare expert (see previous page) just as you would with conventional medical products.

+ Herbal remedies should only be used for a limited amount of time, so seek guidance on duration of use.

+ Seek advice from your doctor or professional therapist before taking herbal remedies if you are taking other medication, are pregnant, breastfeeding, are prone to allergies, have a medical, hormonal, physical, or mental health condition, or for use in the elderly or young.

+ If you are going to have surgery, be aware that herbal remedies can interfere with anesthesia and other medicines used before, during, or after procedures and can interfere with blood-clotting and blood pressure. Always seek medical advice before using.

+ If an herbal remedy causes drowsiness, be mindful about when you use it— avoid use before an activity that requires concentration and focus.

+ Before using herbal remedies for children, always seek professional guidance.

+ Before purchasing your herbal remedy, you might want to check that the manufacturer observes an excellent and legitimate manufacturing process ensuring quality, correct identification, and purity of the plant, as well sustainable sourcing and hygiene.

# USING HERBAL REMEDIES

It is often more effective to combine several herbs together for an enhanced synergetic result. An herbalist can prepare this or you can purchase a ready-made mixture from a naturopathic store or website, but be cautious when purchasing online—make sure to verify authenticity, quality, and sourcing and processing methods. Each part of a plant can have different medicinal uses and the many types of chemical constituents require different extraction methods. Both fresh and dried plant matter are used, depending on the herb. It may take up to 2 weeks before seeing an improvement in sleep, and the dosage level will depend on your sensitivity.

There are several ways to take herbal remedies:

## HERBAL TINCTURE

This is a liquid solution made with a concentrated herbal extract mixed with water and alcohol. Always be guided by your therapist or by the dosage instructions on the packaging, but usually you would take 1-5 ml (1 ml = 20 drops approximately) in a small glass of water, 20 to 30 minutes before bed. More can be taken during the night if needed.

## HERBAL INFUSIONS AND TEAS

Add boiling water to the soft parts of herbs like leaves, flowers, berries, or seeds—just as you would with tea—but infuse for 5 to 15 minutes. Consume as a drink (hot or cold). The general guidance is 1 teaspoon per cup of water. Infusions can also be added to your bath. (For an adult use a small handful and infuse in a pint of water, sieve before adding to the bath water.

## DECOCTION

Simmer the solid or woody part of the plants, such as bark, roots, and seeds, for 10 to 30 minutes, as infusing alone would not be sufficient to extract the beneficial properties. Use 1 teaspoon of the dried herb per cup of water.

## CAPSULES

Taking a capsule, which contains a powder form of the plant, is the simplest way of consuming herbal remedies, especially if you want to avoid drinking too much liquid before bedtime. Consult your herbalist and/or follow the instructions on the packet for the right dosage, which is generally between 400-600 mg per day.

# POPULAR HERBAL REMEDIES TO IMPROVE SLEEP

There are three main categories in terms of properties, but all will help with sleep improvement in some way:

- Calming, relaxing, and balancing the mind.
- Reducing anxiety, heart palpitations and pain, muscle tension, and acting on the nervous system.
- Sedative and sleep-inducing.

In order of popularity:

### LAVENDER *(Lavandula angustifolia or Lavandula officinalis)*
**PROPERTIES**: A great remedy for stress-related problems, lavender helps to calm the nerves, decrease anxious thoughts, and helps you relax and feel ready for sleep. It has a gentle, strengthening effect on the nervous system, and is good for physical and mental exhaustion or when run down.

### CHAMOMILE *(Matricaria recutita)*
**PROPERTIES**: An effective, gentle herb and flower that is calming and soothes away nervous tension, anxiety, restlessness, and hyperactivity. Helps you de-stress and get ready for sleep. Suitable for children and blends well with other herbs.

### VALERIAN *(Valeriana officinalis)*
**PROPERTIES**: Widely used for insomnia and to help release tension, this is a clinically proven sedative with deeply relaxing properties, which also helps to reduce stress, anxiety, and an overactive nervous system. It can help reduce the time to fall asleep. It has antispasmodic properties and helps reduce pain, especially that associated with tension, period pain, colic, and cramps. It should be avoided in case of depression. Combines very well with hops or lemon balm for even better results.

### HOPS *(Humulus lupulus)*
**PROPERTIES**: Used traditionally for insomnia, hops help to reduce tension, anxiety, and restlessness. They have a sedative effect and can make you feel drowsy and help increase sleep duration. Hops combine very well with valerian for better results. Avoid using this remedy if you are prone to depression or breast cancer.

### PASSION FLOWER *(Passiflora incarnata)*
**PROPERTIES**: A traditional herb to help chronic insomnia, especially if associated with stress, tension, and a restless mind. It leaves you feeling refreshed and clear-minded in the morning. It is helpful for the relief of nerve-related pain and twitching limbs. Combined with valerian and hops, or skullcap, it will improve the quality and the quantity of sleep.

LEMON BALM *(Melissa officinalis)*
PROPERTIES: Helps fight stress, insomnia, and promotes healthy sleep. It is advisable to combine lemon balm with other relaxing or sedative herbs, for example in combination with valerian. Lemon balm may interact with the GABA receptors in your brain, which helps to induce sleep.

SKULLCAP *(Scutellaria lateriflora)*
PROPERTIES: A very useful herb for the nerves, skullcap relaxes nervous tension while reviving the central nervous system, when your mind and body are exhausted. It helps calm a restless mind and thoughts at night.

ASHWAGANDHA *(Withania somnifera)*
PROPERTIES: A famous Ayurvedic herb for insomnia, this is traditionally drunk with milk and honey before bedtime. It has a calming yet strengthening effect on the nervous system. It is ideal for someone very active who is prone to exhaustion. Avoid with respiratory conditions.

GERANIUM *(Pelargonium)*
PROPERTIES: Has stress-reducing properties and a sedative effect, which helps you fall back asleep more easily during the night.

SAGE *(Salvia officinalis)*
PROPERTIES: Often available as tablets or a dried tincture, this remedy helps relieve excessive sweating associated with menopausal hot flashes and night sweats, which often disrupt sleep for women. Sage rebalances the sweat-regulating hormones and helps to regulate body temperature.

CALIFORNIA POPPY *(Eschscholzia californica)*
PROPERTIES: One of the more sedative herbs, this can help with excitability of the nervous system, restlessness, and sleeplessness. It also has antispasmodic properties for the relief of pain, cramps, and nerve pain.

WILD LETTUCE *(Lactuca virosa)*
PROPERTIES: Another one of the more sedative herbs available, which is used for insomnia especially if the nervous system is over-active, or in case of excitability, anxiety, restlessness, and for physical stress and muscle pains. Avoid with depression.

LIME BLOSSOM *(Tilia europaea)*
PROPERTIES: Also known as linden or tilia, this is a popular herb for stress, anxiety, and nervous tension.

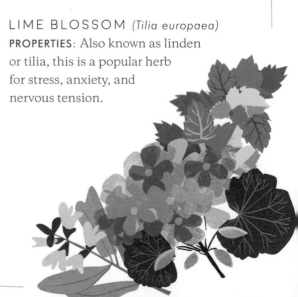

# CHINESE HERBAL REMEDIES

Chinese medicinal herbs and formulas have been used to treat insomnia for over 2,000 years, mostly in China, but also in the Western world relatively recently. The following herbal species are the most prescribed sedative and hypnotic herbs in Chinese herbal medicine. These herbs act through certain neurotransmitters and receptors of the brain and seem to help improve symptoms of insomnia:

**SUANZAOREN DECOCTION**
(*Ziziphus spinosa*): The most frequently used formula

**FULING (*Poria cocos*)**

**GANCAO (*Glycyrrhiza uralensis*)**

**MAGNOLIA BARK (*Magnolia officinalis*):** Used in Asia and in traditional Chinese medicine, this mild sedative may improve sleep by reducing stress, tension, and depression, while lowering anxiety, especially in menopausal women. Its compounds seem to help increase the duration of sleep and lower stress hormones.

# ADAPTOGENS

Adaptogens are herbs, roots, and mushrooms said to protect our central nervous system and our adrenal system against stress and anxiety. They can also help with focus and with endurance when feeling fatigued or weak. They are commonly found in Ayurvedic and traditional Chinese medicine.

The term "adaptogen" was coined by Nikolai Lazarev, a Russian toxicologist, in the late 1940s to describe a plant that helps to adapt to stressful circumstances (mentally, physically, or emotionally). In fact, research shows that adaptogens increase our resilience to stress by putting the body and mind in a state of balance called "homeostasis." They can help our overworked adrenal glands, especially by regulating and balancing stress hormones. Adaptogens for sleep include:

**AMERICAN GINSENG (*Panax quinquefolius*):** Enhances cognitive function, but is less stimulating than Asian ginseng and a better option for the relief of anxiety.

**ASHWAGANDHA (*Withania somnifera*):** Effectively reduces stress and anxiety by decreasing the stress hormone cortisol and improving how your body responds to stress. It generally also helps with depression and insomnia. Avoid with respiratory conditions.

**RHODIOLA (*Rhodiola rosea*):** Combats stress, protects cellular and metabolic function from prolonged exposure to chronic stress, and prevents chronic fatigue. It also has antidepressant properties by balancing neurotransmitters in the brain. Avoid with high blood pressure and nervous conditions.

# CBD PRODUCTS

CBD, also known as cannabidiol, is extracted from the stalk, leaves, stems, and flowers of the hemp plant and has no psychoactive effects ("high") associated with it, unlike THC, another well-known cannabinoid. CBD products seem to help reduce anxiety, stress, insomnia, pain, and improve mental focus upon waking. CBD can apparently make you feel relaxed and serene and help you to fall asleep faster. It is proven by research that CBD supports the natural sleep–wake cycles, helping you to sleep for longer durations and helping you to stay more alert during the day when used in small doses. To be approved, these products cannot have a THC content higher than 0.2 percent.

According to the World Health Organization "CBD is generally well tolerated with a good safety profile . . . To date, there is no evidence of recreational use of CBD or any public health-related problems associated with the use of pure CBD." That said, clinical studies are ongoing to understand the effects of CBD on a wide range of conditions.

CBD is not addictive, but it responds differently depending on your sensitivity to the substance. In fact, this product is available in a variety of different concentration and strength levels. For the purest form of this product, opt for organic products that use a $CO_2$ extraction method. CBD is available as:

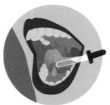

**SUBLINGUAL OIL:** Spray or place drops under the tongue and hold there for 20 to 60 seconds before swallowing. Increase the dosage progressively depending on the concentration levels and your tolerance level. It is best to start with a very low dose and increase gradually, until you find something that works for you. As an indication, you can use 5-70 mg per day.

**CAPSULES:** Opt for capsules if you want to avoid the strong flavour of CBD.

**EDIBLE CBD SWEETS:** Opt for sweets if you want to lessen the strong flavour of CBD.

**BALMS:** Rub a small amount onto the skin. Balms are also effective for pain management when rubbed into the affected area.

**MASSAGE OILS AND LOTIONS:** A massage performed with CBD-infused oils (CBD oil incorporated and diluted into a carrier oil) is claimed to have effective relaxation properties, calming inflammation, and reducing anxiety, tension, and chronic pain.

**E-LIQUIDS:** CBD e-liquids can be used in e-cigarettes and inhaled; this gives the highest absorption rate.

# FLOWER ESSENCES

Flower essences are also therapeutic, but they are different from herbal medicine or aromatherapy, because the healing powers come from the flowers' energetic rather than physical properties. They tackle the emotional states and issues that prevent us from achieving balance and well-being. Similarly to aromatherapy (see pages 171–175), choosing the best flower essences for your sleep is a combination of your intuition and of knowledge about their properties, which a practitioner can help you with. The most popular flower essences are Dr. Bach's Flower Remedies and Australian Bush Flower Essences.

## HOW THEY ARE CREATED

The "sun" method involves placing the flowers into spring water and leaving them to stand in the sun for several hours to capture the flowers' energy into the water. The water is later mixed with a grape alcohol solution to preserve the essence. An alternative method for certain flowers, however, is to first simmer them in spring water for 30 minutes, and then proceed to the "sun" method.

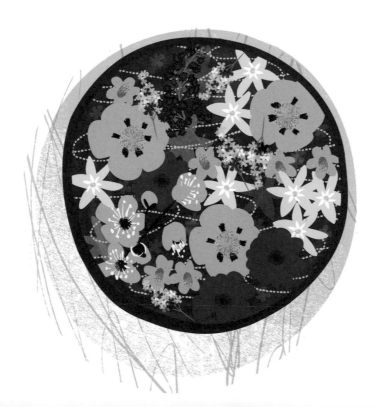

## HOW THEY ARE USED

The recommendation is to use 2–7 drops several times a day by mixing with water and drinking, or using pure drops underneath the tongue. Or you can create a spray mix with some water. Follow the instructions on the packaging and be aware that it will take a few weeks to feel the results.

There are 38 flowers. The most popular flower essences for sleep are:

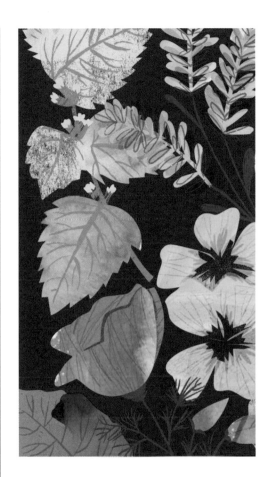

+ **WHITE CHESTNUT (*Aesculus Hippocastanum*):** For help with rumination and restlessness.
+ **RED HORSE-CHESTNUT (*Aesculus carnea*):** To feel calmer, worry less, and feel more confident, reassured, and peaceful.
+ **ASPEN (*Populus tremula*):** For anxious feelings.
+ **MIMULUS (*Mimulus guttatus*):** To face your fears.
+ **VERVAIN (*Verbena officinalis*):** To calm down when overstimulated.
+ **STAR OF BETHLEHEM (*Ornithogalum umbellatum*):** To heal from trauma, sadness, and shock.
+ **CHERRY PLUM (*Prunus cerasifera*):** Helps with fear of losing control, when you are the verge of a breakdown, or in despair or feeling angry.
+ **IMPATIENS (*Impatiens glandulifera*):** For when you feel irritable, tense, and fidgety.
+ **ROCK ROSE (*Helianthemum*):** For frozen terror and panic.
+ **RED SUVA FRANGIPANI (*Plumeria ruba*):** For when you want to feel calm and nurtured, and have inner peace and strength to cope.

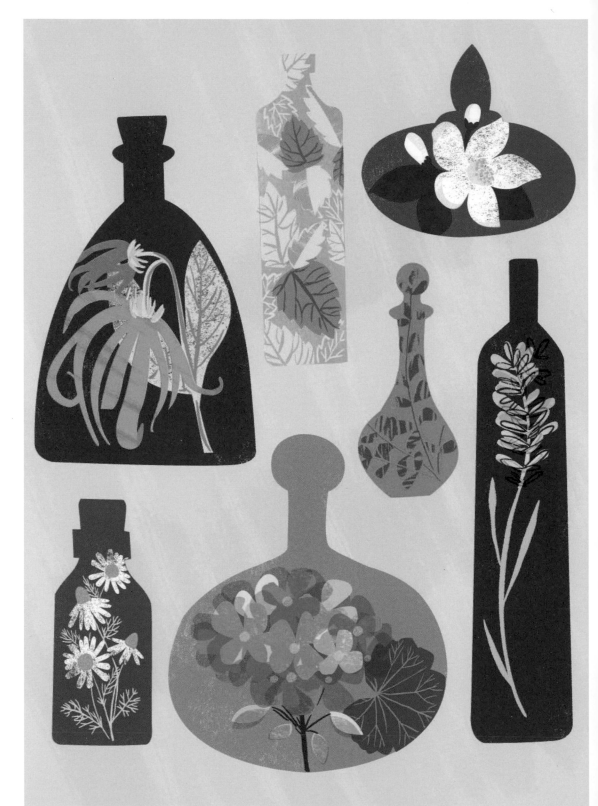

# AROMATHERAPY

Aromatherapy is a complementary therapy based on the sense of smell of pure essential oils to heal the body and mind. While it can't cure chronic insomnia, it can ease your ability to drift off to sleep by making you feel more relaxed and less anxious. It is important to trust your intuition and immediate gut reaction to a scent to find out what suits you best. The effect can be felt almost instantly. Be aware of the safety guidelines (see page 172) before using essential oils.

## USING AROMATHERAPY OILS

You can either inhale essential oils through your nose or apply them as a topical application on your skin—thanks to their transdermal properties, the oils will enter your bloodstream. While combining oils can be effective, mixing more than seven oils is not recommended as it could be detrimental and the oils may lose their potency. An aromatherapist can advise you about choosing essential oils, including how much to use and how to blend them.

The oils of your choice can be used in several ways. For example:

BATHTIME: Add up to 5 drops of pure essential oil to your bath water.

BEDTIME: Sprinkle or spray a couple of drops of pure essential oil on your pillowcase from 30 minutes to an hour before bedtime, or spray onto a handkerchief and place it near your head. To make a pillow spray, add the oil to a bit of water in a mini spray bottle or you can purchase ready-made pillow sprays too.

MASSAGE: Rub into a specific body part (feet, wrists, palms, chest, neck, shoulders, scalp, temples). You can use a couple of drops directly on your skin as long as you have done the skin patch test (see page 172) and aren't being exposed to direct sunlight. But it is much safer to use a diluted version, adding 10 drops of pure essential oil to about 20 ml of carrier oil (sweet almond, argan, jojoba, unscented coconut, grapeseed, sunflower).

# SAFETY FIRST

- Make sure you blow out candles before bedtime.

- Make sure not to leave a lit candle underneath an oil burner bowl if the water is fully evaporated, or else the burner may crack.

- Seek advice from your physician or professional therapist before using aromatherapeutic remedies, particularly if you are taking other medication, are pregnant, breastfeeding, on medication, allergy prone, or have a serious or chronic medical or mental condition, or for use in the elderly or young.

- Check with your physician before taking aromatherapeutic remedies if you are going to have surgery or have any respiratory condition.

- Dilute the oil in a carrier oil and do a skin patch test to prevent any allergic or photosensitive reactions. The latter means that UV rays could cause permanent marks on your skin. Do a patch test, usually on the inside of your wrist or arm, and then wait for 24 to 48 hours to observe any reaction or sensitivity.

- Never use essential oils on any mucous membrane, such as inside the mouth or the nose.

- Some oils can be ingested, but never do so without seeking professional advice.

- Use organic oils labeled as pure or 100 percent essential oil and make sure the Latin name is given for each plant to guarantee it is not a synthetic oil.

- If use of an oil causes drowsiness, be mindful about when you use it—avoid use before an activity that requires concentration and focus.

- Before using essential oils for children, always seek professional guidance.

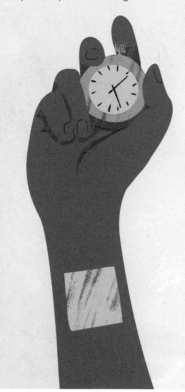

SMELL: Dilute in an unscented carrier oil and then rub into your hands, and smell the scent with several deep breaths.

PULSE POINTS ROLL-ONS OR BALMS: Rub your aromatherapy roll-on stick or creamy balm on your pulse points in a slow circular motion for 5 to 10 seconds on the inside of your wrist, and on your temples. There are seven pulse points on the body, such as the ankles and neck, but the wrists and temples are the most accessible ones for aromatherapy. Once applied, inhale the aroma in two or three deep breaths through your nose, and out through your mouth.

AROMATHERAPY CANDLES: Candles provide lovely dim lighting, a relaxing ambience, and can also help you sleep with relaxing and therapeutic scents. Make sure you blow out your candles before falling asleep and never leave unattended. Avoid paraffin or synthetic wax candles as they can release harmful by-products. Instead, choose organic beeswax or soy wax candles with an organic cotton wick (unbleached and uncoated). Ensure that your chosen candle is made with pure organic essential essential oils, as opposed to synthetic fragrances.

OIL BURNERS: These facilitate the diffusion of pure essential oils into your bedroom. First, fill the burner bowl with a small amount of water and add 3–5 drops of pure essential oil(s) into the

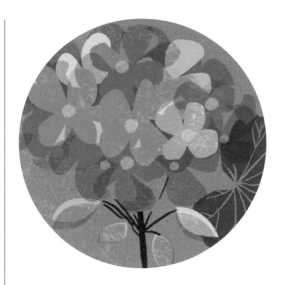

water. Then place a lit tealight candle underneath the bowl to heat the water, which will release the scent of the oil(s) as the mixture gently evaporates. To clean your oil burner, wipe the bowl with a paper towel then wash with soap and water.

ROOM DIFFUSER: Add 5 drops of essential oil to your room diffuser; it is generally mixed with a bit of water, but always be guided by the packet instructions. The diffuser should automatically shut down once empty.

INHALATION: Pour 4 cups of boiling water into a heat-resistant bowl then add up to 10 drops of pure essential oil. Place your face on top of it with a towel over your head, allowing the steam to rise into your nostrils and inhale deeply.

# ESSENTIAL OILS FOR GOOD SLEEP

Essential oils for sleep can be categorized as follows:

- Sleep-inducing oils that calm the mind and reduce anxiety symptoms.
- Oils that clear the airways to facilitate breathing and prevent snoring.

Here are the oils in order of popularity:

### ENGLISH LAVENDER
(Lavandula angustifolia)
**PROPERTIES**: One of the most renowned oils for sleep, lavender has a harmonizing effect on the nervous system, lifting or calming as needed. It is one of the best oils for helping cope with stress and mild insomnia. Note that using too much lavender essential oil can be stimulating rather than sedating—a few drops on a piece of fabric is sufficient.

### ROMAN CHAMOMILE
(Anthemis nobilis)
**PROPERTIES**: Soothing, calming, and an antidepressant, Roman chamomile in particular is excellent for relieving stress, anxiety, irritability, and nervous tension that can lead to insomnia. It's a gentle oil and is suitable for children over six months of age after consulting with a pediatrician and doing a patch test.

### CLARY SAGE (Salvia sclarea)
**PROPERTIES**: This sleep-inducing oil is beneficial in relieving stress, nervous tension, anxiety, and in fighting depression. It helps balance and also relax and has a tonic effect for nervous and mental fatigue and gives tranquility and feelings of well-being. Be mindful of when you use this oil, as it can cause drowsiness in some people.

### SWEET MARJORAM
(Origanum majorana)
**PROPERTIES**: This has the ability to both strengthen and relax the nerves and is recommended for nervous tension and when you are unable to relax, but feel fatigued and have stress-related insomnia. It can be strongly sedative and cause you to feel drowsy so be mindful of when you use it. It may reduce sexual impulse.

### VETIVER (Chrysopogon zizanioides or Vetiveria zizanioides)
**PROPERTIES**: A relaxing oil, this is beneficial for stress, anxiety, insomnia, and depression. It's recommended for physical and emotional burnout or for being overwhelmed from exhaustion and being under pressure. It has a grounding, centering effect, helping with meditation and calming the mind. It can also give effective pain relief.

### NEROLI (Citrus aurantium amara)
**PROPERTIES**: Regarded as one of the most effective sedative and antidepressant essential oils, also useful for the treatment of insomnia and anxiety, neroli

is good for someone who is emotionally intense and easily alarmed and agitated. It promotes calm and stability, aids sleep, helps clear the mind, and lift spirits.

YLANG YLANG (Cananga odorata)
PROPERTIES: Known for its ability to slow down rapid breathing and calm the palpitations often associated with anxiety and anger, this has a sedating and calming effect and is helpful as an antidepressant oil, for calming frustration, stress, tension, anxiety, panic, and insomnia.

LEMON BALM (Melissa officinalis)
PROPERTIES: Helps fight stress, insomnia, and promotes healthy sleep. It is recommended to combine lemon balm with other relaxing or sedative herbs. Lemon balm may interact with the GABA receptors in your brain that help to induce sleep.

GERANIUM (Pelargonium)
PROPERTIES: Its stress-reducing properties help you fall back asleep more easily during the night. It is known to help treat restlessness, anxiety, palpitations, and panic attacks. Useful for people who wake up during the night and feel panicky and hot. Some claim it also has a sedative effect.

CARDAMOM (Elettaria cardamomum)
PROPERTIES: An essential oil that calms and clears the mind, this is a gentle tonic of the nervous system and recommended

for times of nervous exhaustion and depression. It's ideal for someone burdened by worries and responsibilities.

FRANKINCENSE (Boswellia sacra)
PROPERTIES: Helps alleviate anxiety, nervous tension, and stress-related conditions such as insomnia, irritability, and restlessness. It is a useful aid to meditation, helping calm mental chatter and quietening the mind.

MANDARIN (Citrus reticulata)
PROPERTIES: Known as a children's essential oil, but effective for adults, too, this is helpful for calming restlessness and hyperactivity, and also for soothing stress, anxiety, nervous tension, and tackling insomnia.

BERGAMOT (Citrus bergamia)
PROPERTIES: Extracted from a fruit that is like a mix between lemon and orange, this essence is known to reduce anxiety and stress and has antidepressant properties because it is both calming and invigorating. It is also known for helping relax muscle tension, spasm, and can help clear respiratory airways.

ORANGE (Citrus sinensis)
PROPERTIES: Has a calming effect on the digestive system and calms any nervous tension, helps lift depression, and facilitates sleep.

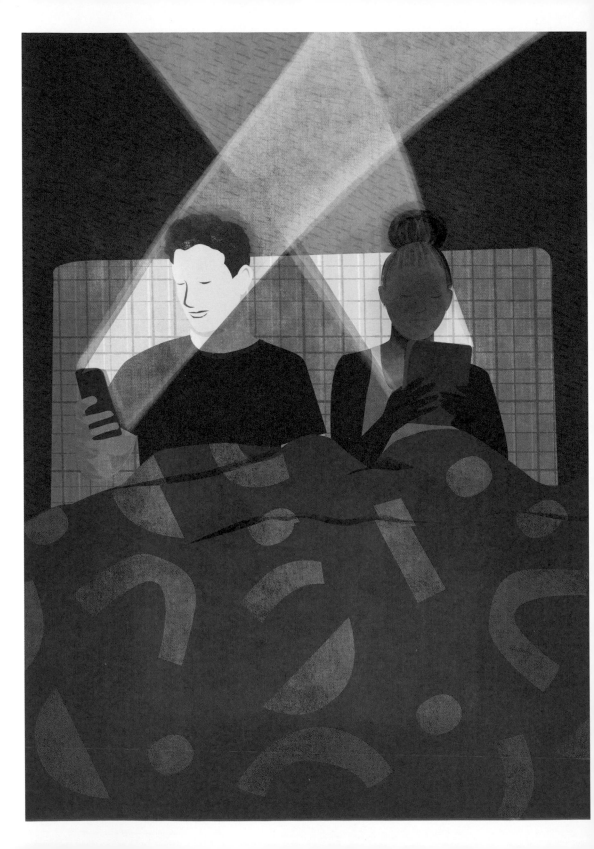

# SLEEP TECH

Sleep technology can be our sleep friend or sleep enemy, depending on how and what it is used for. Using technology in the hope that it will solve any sleep issues overnight with no effort on our part might be unrealistic, but combining technology with other natural solutions and techniques, along with a regular digital detox practice, might just work for you. Sleep tech can help us monitor and optimize our sleep, help us experiment with sensory and relaxing experiences, and give us added support in our quest for better sleep.

## FINDING WHAT WORKS FOR YOU

Once your relationship with technology becomes healthy and measured rather than obsessive or addictive, then you can use it responsibly and explore an exciting range of gadgets that can support your sleep (even if it only gives you the illusion that it does, that is good enough!).

Some, but not all, sleep tech is backed by scientific studies—ultimately, what matters is finding a solution that inspires you and works for you.

## A HYPERCONNECTED LIFESTYLE

Receiving ongoing alerts, emails, notifications, and digital content overstimulates very specific areas of our brain. It captivates and holds our focus for extended durations and can give a false sense of danger or excitement, preventing us from sleeping soundly. Devices that track and monitor our sleep can create performance anxiety and unnecessary worries, also robbing us of a good night's sleep. Checking our devices and personal data for updates frequently, sometimes as often as every 5 to 10 minutes, feeds our fear of missing out (FOMO) and creates an ongoing sense of alert and vigilance not conducive to a relaxed state of mind.

### AN ALERT BRAIN

So why are our gadgets so hard to ignore or resist? Why are they so addictive? This is how the brain responds to a hyperconnected lifestyle:

1. Notifications and alerts stimulate the parietal lobe, auditory cortex, and visual cortex, which make up our brain's attention and alert system. As a comparison, imagine if your doorbell rang, then stopped, then started again, all day long. How would you feel at the end of the day? Stressed? Waiting for the next ring?

2. Rewarding and instant gratification features such as "like," "comment," and "click here for" stimulate the ventral tegmental area of the brain, which then releases the popular and addictive neurotransmitter dopamine, giving the feeling of pleasure. The easier it is to get your reward, the more likely you are to repeat a behavior compulsively. A study showed that activating this part of a rat's brain led it to push on the stimulation lever until it was close to dying.[1]

3. Binge-watching a continuous playlist of videos or TV episodes, with the autoplay feature and a countdown to the next episode, immerses the brain into a state of "flow." This means total immersion in and concentration on never-ending content, fooling the visual cortex in the brain into not understanding limits and boundaries, in addition to engaging the brain's reward system with instant gratification.

4. Talking about yourself on social media and receiving social acknowledgment, praise, and invitations results in a stimulation cocktail for the brain, releasing dopamine and engaging with the precuneus, the area of the brain that also deals with self-awareness and self-consciousness and with the inferior frontal gyrus, which handles language processing and production.

5. Disconnecting from your daily digital tools and platforms or losing your smartphone creates deep anxiety about missing out, which activates the amygdala, the part of the brain that plays a primary role in emotional responses such as fear, anxiety, and aggression.

## DIGITAL DETOX

To start a new digital detox habit:

+ Consider stopping the use of brain-stimulating and light-emitting devices at least 2 to 4 hours before bedtime, especially if this might result in disturbing interactions or thoughts.
+ Be aware of how having gadgets in the bedroom will affect the ambience of your bedroom (see Building a Cocoon, pages 52–63).
+ If you have gadgets in your bedroom, turn the sound, lights, and notifications off, and be disciplined about not checking them during the night.
+ Make incremental changes, one at a time, little by little. For example, if not having your phone in your bedroom feels too difficult, try putting it in a drawer to begin with. Remember, it takes 21 days on average to change a habit.
+ Or take a more radical approach by moving yourself outside of your daily life and become immersed in a brand-new environment fostering sleep, such as a sleep retreat, a digital

detox retreat, or a mind, body, and soul vacation with yoga and meditation.

# RESPIRATORY AIDS AND ANTI-SNORING DEVICES

During sleep, snoring might not be an issue if it is relatively mild, but heavy snoring and obstructive sleep apnea (OSA) can be a cause for concern. These conditions are caused either by a collapse of the soft tissues in the back of the throat and tongue, a softening of the upper airways' muscle tone, or a blockage in the nose often due to a deviated septum (the thin wall between your nasal passages is off center), any of which can obstruct the respiratory passages and make breathing difficult. Not breathing properly while sleeping can lead to high blood pressure, cardiovascular diseases, mood disorders, and low energy, as well as concentration and memory issues.

The best way to work out whether you need might need a respiratory aid is if someone notices that you breathe very loudly or, worse, regularly stop breathing during the night, or gasp for air, even if it is for just a moment. OSA and heavy snoring impact on the deep sleep quality for both the sufferer and their bed partner.

Before turning to technology, there are some natural ways you can help yourself too. For starters, it is important to drink enough water and lubricate your airways and reduce dryness in your nose and throat. It is wise to increase muscle tone in the airways with tongue and throat exercises which you can discuss with your respiratory expert.[2] Any respiratory devices should also be supplemented by lifestyle changes, as needed, such as weight loss, quitting smoking, and avoiding alcohol. Sleeping on your side (rather than on your back) is the best option for most snorers, this will prevent your fully relaxed tongue from lodging itself in the back of the throat although it may not help people who are overweight or obese. For more serious cases, surgery might be an option.

## CONTINUOUS POSITIVE AIRWAY PRESSURE (CPAP) DEVICE

This is the most popular device to treat sleep apnea. It pumps air into the nose and/or mouth adjusting the air pressure as needed, but it is a beast of a device that covers the face, which can feel uncomfortable while sleeping.

There are lighter alternatives for less serious cases; some of these are vented, while others are meant to be positioned either on the bottom of your face or on your nostrils in a way that lets the air in.

## VENTED OR NON-VENTED FACE AND NOSE MASKS

This headgear is adjusted around the front of the face and the back of the head with a breathing aid.

## MOUTHGUARDS (MANDIBULAR DEVICES)

These position the mouth, lower jaw, and tongue to leave an open airway passage during the night.

## CHIN STRAPS

These straps may help you sleep better by holding your mouth closed and thereby preventing open-mouth snoring, but they should not be used if your nose is blocked.

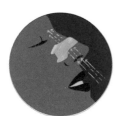

## LIPS OR NASAL ADHESIVE STRIPS

+ **FOR THE NOSE**: These disposable clear plastic adhesive strips are worn over the bridge of the nose, lifting and opening up the nasal passages and improving airflow.
+ **FOR THE MOUTH**: These strips are applied to the lips instead, and have a small opening for mouth breathing.

## SMART SNORING DETECTORS

These sleep gadgets are placed underneath the pillow or built into a smart pillow, which automatically detects when you're snoring and then gently moves your head or vibrates to prevent further snoring.

# SLEEP DIAGNOSTIC AND TRACKING TOOLS

Data-driven sleep-tracking tools are useful to get a rough idea of sleep patterns and observe overall trends, but be aware that they are often inaccurate. Do not become obsessive or concerned by your "results" because of perfectionist tendencies and goals you couldn't "achieve."

## WEARABLES AND SMARTPHONES

Personal smart watches, wrist devices, and smartphones have built-in apps that are meant to measure your sleep duration, cycles, heart rate, and overnight awakenings as part of your daily activity tracking. There is also a wearable ring that measures pulse, heart rate variability, movements, and body temperature with built-in sensors. The tracking with these devices isn't entirely accurate because it is not based on brain waves and other biofeedback

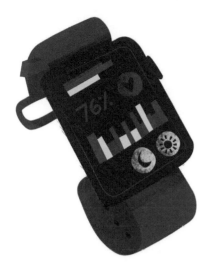

measurements. At best, it might be a loose indicator of your sleep, so you should not obsess over the results.

## CONTACT-FREE SLEEP MONITORS

These sensors provide sleep-tracking data without the need to wear a tracking device. You can find them as bedside sensors or as pads placed under the pillow, sheets, or mattress. In addition to monitoring sleep, many provide additional data such as breathing patterns while sleeping (including snoring and apnea), heart rate (including variability), bedroom temperature, environmental sound, light level, and humidity.

## SMART TRACKING DEVICES

These devices use electroencephalogram (EEG) technology to measure the electrical activity of the brain, tracking

and recording brain-wave patterns. Some products respond to the sleep data and deliver technological solutions to help improve it:

+ **HEAD BANDS AND SMART HEADPHONES WITH BUILT-IN EEG CAPABILITIES**: These devices have sensors that measure and detect brain waves. Some models are designed to respond by emitting noise patterns, vibrations, frequencies, or guided meditations through built-in speakers, slowing down brain waves and helping extend and improve deep sleep in particular. This headgear usually comes in the form of headphones, a headband, or a headset.

+ **BIOFEEDBACK SYSTEMS**: Biofeedback and neurofeedback techniques (see pages 134–138) help you learn how to control some of your body's functions. With these devices you are connected to electrical sensors that help you receive real-time information about your body such as pulse rate, pulse strength, heart rate variability (HRV), brain waves, body temperature, breathing, and muscle tension. They can also give you a real-time display of trends, guidance on your breathing, and an evaluation of how relaxed you are. These sensors can be built into wearables headsets, or simply plugged into your connected device with a companion app.

# SMART LIGHTING

Nothing can replace natural lighting when it comes to impacting our sleep-wake cycles, yet when sleep becomes difficult it is worth exploring light therapy (see pages 69-71). Smart lighting in the form of tech devices emitting or blocking artificial light can help you achieve better sleep. Here are a few for your consideration:

## WAKE-UP LIGHTING

Bedside alarm clocks with morning lighting and sound options help you wake up by imitating the natural light from a sunrise. The aim is to make you feel ready and energized, rather than startled upon awakening. The luminosity increases gradually about 30 minutes before your desired wake-up time. It stimulates a more gentle and gradual release of hormones responsible for waking you up and suppresses your sleep hormone. Some of these devices are also medically certified to treat SAD (seasonal affective disorder) and have features such as radio, USB, and Bluetooth connections for sound, or even differentiated evening and morning light color.

## LIGHT PULSATOR

This device projects a pulsating light on the ceiling. Synchronizing your breath to the visual pulsations, in such a way that you exhale twice as long as you inhale, seems to facilitate sleep onset.

## SEASONAL AFFECTIVE DISORDER (SAD) LIGHTING

Some people who struggle with SAD or have a circadian rhythm disorder (see page 37) can improve their mood and sleep by exposing themselves to a SAD light box for 30 minutes to an hour every morning. The intensity of the light is measured in lux (units of illumination) and research shows bright light of 2,500 lux improves well-being. Indoor illumination is 300-500 lux, whereas outdoor light varies from 1,500 lux on a cloudy day up to 120,000 lux on a sunny day. Don't use a SAD light if you have an eye condition or eye damage, and avoid evening use as it will suppress the natural release of your sleep hormone.

## BLUE-LIGHT FILTERS

As explained on pages 66-67, blue light emitted from electronic device screens in the evening may confuse your brain into thinking it is daytime. Too much blue light can impact your circadian rhythm or damage your eyesight, but some research also shows that it plays a relatively small role in increasing sleep duration and quality. That said, it's a good thing to signal wind-down time to your brain by lowering the light levels and decreasing exposure to blue light.

+ Switch on the dark or night mode wherever available on gadgets.
+ Use a blue filter app such as f.lux or Twilight. These make the screen color and brightness of your computers, tablets, and smartphones adapt to the time of day, gradually decreasing the shiny bright blue light late afternoon and increasing warm amber red tones from late afternoon onward. It is recommended to let the light automatically dim down to even deeper tones from 2 to 4 hours before bedtime. It is also key not to increase your screen's brightness to compensate for the lack of blue light, otherwise it defeats the purpose.
+ Try wearing blue-light-filter eyeglasses. Although not endorsed by everyone in the medical profession, it is claimed that they can block blue light if you work at a screen all day long and can be as stylish as regular glasses.
+ Traditional eye masks reinvented in the form of specialty eye masks with padded eye contours create an entirely blackout effect even when your eyes are open underneath. There are also eye masks with built-in hypnotic lights designed to send you off to sleep.
+ Dimmer switches, dimmable light

bulbs, and blue-light-free bulbs are simple solutions to create cosy evening lighting, and facilitate your wind-down before sleep.

# APPS FOR CONNECTED SMART DEVICES

Once you are in control of your smart device "addiction," it's a good idea to explore the world of apps, and know the ones that can support your quest for better sleep. There are many useful apps that can either relax, monitor, or help with sleep.

### MEDITATION

As explained in the Taming the Mind (see pages 86–95) and Beditation (see pages 74–85) sections, meditation and mindfulness are an amazing off switch for our brains and bodies and, an excellent way to support your mental health and sleep. There are hundreds of meditation apps on the market. Here are some of the most popular ones:

+ **CALM:** Guided meditation and relaxation, celebrity sleep stories, calming sounds, and podcasts.
+ **HEADSPACE:** Guided and group meditation, soothing sounds, exercise, and inspirational talks.
+ **LIBERATE:** Meditation app for the

Black, Indigenous, and People of Color communities.

+ **AURA**: Mindfulness and meditation app for stress, anxiety, and sleep.
+ **BUDDHIFY**: Guided meditations adapted to your day.
+ **PZIZZ**: Bedtime/naptime meditations, soundscapes, and voice-overs.
+ **INSCAPE**: Personalized mindfulness, breathing and meditation sessions.
+ **UNPLUG MEDITATION**: Popular guided meditation videos.

## SLEEP TRACKING

Many devices have a built-in activity tracker (see page 181), but there are also standalone activity tracking apps:

+ **SLEEP CYCLE ALARM**: This sleep analysis app monitors your sleep and wakes you with an alarm when you are in your lightest sleep pattern.
+ **SLEEPSCORE**: Provides sleep analysis, optimized wake-up alarm, information, and advice.
+ **OTHER POPULAR BUILT-IN ACTIVITY TRACKING APPS**: Fitbit, Health Mate (Withings, Nokia), Activity (Apple Watch), Samsung Health.
+ **CHECKY**: This app (by Calm) calculates the number of times you checked your smartphone every day so you can monitor your smartphone "addiction."

## SOUNDS

+ **SLEEP SOLUTIONS**: Complex new scientific sound technology, combining multiple techniques and processes for sleep, stress, well-being and performance—a sort of therapeutic "sonic massage."
+ **SONIC SLEEP**: Uses a phone's microphone to assess background noise and then employs an AI-powered algorithm to pick out the right audio to mask it.
+ **MOSHI TWILIGHT SLEEP STORIES**: Bedtime stories, music, and nighttime themes aimed at sending kids to sleep.
+ **CALM**: Meditation, as well as sleep stories read by celebrities, calming music, and sounds.

## SLEEP CALCULATORS

Some apps can calculate the time at which you should go to sleep based on the time you intend to wake up, generally based on a 90-minute sleep cycle.

+ **SLEEPYTI.ME**
+ **SLEEP CALCULATOR**

## CBTI

While it has been clinically proven to be effective, implementing cognitive behavioral therapy for insomnia (see page 88) can be difficult on your own. There are apps with interactive courses available to help guide you, but you may also want to seek professional advice.

+ **SLEEPSTATION** (UK, free with the NHS through a referral scheme)
+ **SLEEPIO** (UK, US through CVS Health)
+ **CBTI COACH** (UK)
+ **SOMRYST** (US)

## SNORING

+ **SOUNDLY**: Exercises to reduce snoring.
+ **SLEEP.AI**: Claims to detect sleep apnea, snoring, and teeth-grinding by analyzing sound samples, and works with an anti-snore wearable claimed to stop you from snoring.

# SOUND DEVICES FOR SLEEP

In Sound Asleep (see pages 149–159), we learn how sounds can help us improve our sleep duration and quality. Fortunately, there are sleep-friendly sound devices used to cover up sudden, loud, or repetitive noises, and also to play sounds and frequencies likely to make us feel relaxed and send us into slumber. So how can you block disruptive noises or listen to healing sounds while sleeping?

## HEADPHONES AND EARBUDS

Sleep-speciliazed headphones and ear buds are optimized for comfortable sleeping, especially lying on your side. There are many to choose from with differing levels of comfort and sound quality, and depending on your budget.

+ Earbuds (inserted in the ear openings), headphones (sit on top of your ears), fabric headband-style headphones (sit around your forehead and head), and headset-style phones (sit on top of your head and ears).
+ Some have features such as noise-cancellation, noise-masking, responsive EEG tracking, and features showing you how to control your brain waves.
+ Often hearing devices use a combination of active and passive noise cancelation in addition to sounds. Passive means creating a block between the noisy environment and the ear canal, whereas active noise cancelation (ANC) has the net effect of canceling out any environmental noise by processing audio signals in a specific way.
+ Fabric headbands can have built-in earphones or mini speakers either wired or connected via Bluetooth to your smartphone and have volume/pause/play controls.

## PILLOW SPEAKERS

These stereo speakers, either wired or connected via Bluetooth, have volume control either built into the pillows or placed under your existing pillow.

You can enjoy your favorite music or sounds for optimal relaxation and comfort by connecting them to an audio device.

## FREQUENCY-EMITTING DEVICES AND WHITE NOISE MACHINES

Frequency-emitting devices generate frequencies that slow down your brain waves from alpha (awake state) to theta (light sleep) to delta (deeper sleep), helping you relax and fall asleep.

White-noise machines can play a range of noise-masking and relaxation sounds and frequencies for better sleep. Some have adaptive capabilities by reacting to the environmental sound levels and adjusting the volume accordingly. You can set a timer so it shuts off automatically. Portable mini versions are also available for travel. Some of these machines are also optimized to relieve tinnitus (perceived sound with ears ringing at a very high pitch). See also pages 151–152 for more about white noise.

# TEXTILE PRODUCTS

What you sleep "in" matters just as much as what you sleep "on" for a good night's sleep. It is therefore worth exploring these textile-based products as a simple way to support your sleep.

## THERMO-REGULATED SLEEPWEAR AND BEDDING

Feeling too cold or too hot during the night, especially getting hot flashes during the menopausal years for women, is quite common and can prevent a good night's sleep. After adjusting your bedroom and bedding temperature to an adequate level (see pages 55–61), consider purchasing thermo-regulated sleepwear and bedding made with adaptive textiles and materials that self-adjust to the body's changing temperature. They provide better sleep comfort by combining evaporation and moisture-wicking technology to keep you cool.

## WEIGHTED SLEEP PRODUCTS

+ **EYE PILLOWS**: These cases filled with beads or seeds rest on your eyes for a moment of relaxation and to give acupressure around the eyes. Sometimes infused with aromatic oils or dried herbs, eye pillows can relieve headaches, insomnia, and eye strain.
+ **WEIGHTED BLANKETS**: Reported to help release serotonin, oxytocin, and dopamine, and keep your nervous system calm by simulating the feeling of being held, weighted blankets apparently reduce nighttime anxieties and help release the sleep hormone melatonin and reduce the stress hormone cortisol. The theory is that acupressure distributes the weight and

pressure evenly across your body while keeping you cool.

# SLEEP AND RELAXATION PODS

If you need a moment of deep relaxation or napping on the go, you may want to try these "hi tech" cocoons designed to help you rest and recover. These seem futuristic and unusual, but tech-savvy enthusiasts might find in them just what they need to help manage their daytime energy levels.

## NAP PODS AND NAP STATIONS

An increasing number of businesses offer pods where employees and visitors can take a restorative nap during work hours. Such pods or stations can also be found in various pop-up locations and in airports. The pods look like capsules and have a comfortable reclining chair or a flat bed protected by an overhead screen, curtains, sliding door or roller blinds, which can be closed for privacy.

## FLOATING THERAPY TANKS

Also called sensory deprivation tanks, these are large private enclosed cubicles filled with salted water in which you can float at a comfortable temperature, enveloped in darkness and silence or with dimmed lights and music. This floating experience is meant to relieve tension in the body, calm the nervous system and provide a moment of relaxation. Results may carry through to a more peaceful night's sleep.

# BEDROOM ENVIRONMENT

These products are designed to enhance our environment for better sleep.

## AIR PURIFIERS

As mentioned on page 56, it is important to optimize your bedroom's air quality. Air purifiers come in very handy for this as they remove pollutants, allergens, and particles from the air with an advanced filtration system.

## SMART BEDS

Technologically advanced beds and mattresses are engineered for more comfort and better sleep. Responsive technology with internal sensors adjusts the mattress to the optimum temperature, firmness, and support. Some track sleep data and can provide a virtual sleep coach app that delivers sleep insights and recommendations based on your sleep history.

# INDEX

# ENDNOTES AND SOURCES

## INTRODUCTION AND UNDERSTANDING SLEEP (PAGES 6–37)

1. CDC: *https://www.cdc.gov/sleep/data_statistics.html*
2. NSF: *https://www.sleepfoundation.org/sleep-disorders/insomnia*
3. "Why sleep matters—the economic costs of insufficient sleep: A cross-country comparative analysis." RAND Corporation, 2016.
4. Neuroscience research center in Lyon, France.
5. "Trends in Outpatient Visits for Insomnia, Sleep Apnea, and Prescriptions for Sleep Medications among US Adults: Findings from the National Ambulatory Medical Care Survey 1999–2010,' *Sleep*, Volume 37, Issue 8, 1 August 2014, Pages 1283–1293, *https://doi.org/10.5665/sleep.3914 https://academic.oup.com/sleep/article/37/8/1283/2416804*
6. "Evidence for the Efficacy of Melatonin in the Treatment of Primary Adult Sleep Disorders." *Sleep Medicine Reviews*, 2017. *https://pubmed.ncbi.nlm.nih.gov/28648359/*

## WIND-DOWN PRACTICES AND RITUALS (PAGES 40–51)

1. "Beauty sleep: experimental study on the perceived health and attractiveness of sleep deprived people." (2010) *https://www.ncbi.nlm.nih.gov/pubmed/21156746*
2. *https://www.sleep.org/articles/washing-your-face-before-bed/*

## BUILDING YOUR COCOON (PAGES 52–63)

1. A. K. Mishra's research from the Eindhoven University of Technology, the Netherlands—"Window/door opening-mediated bedroom ventilation and its impact on sleep quality of healthy, young adults." (2017)
2. *https://www.psychologytoday.com/gb/blog/canine-corner/201709/should-you-let-your-dog-sleep-in-bed-you*
3. New study, led by Laurence Bayer and Sophie Schwartz, University of Geneva, Switzerland. Perrault et al. "Whole-Night Continuous Rocking Entrains Spontaneous Neural Oscillations with Benefits for Sleep and Memory." *Current Biology*, DOI: 10.1016/j.cub.2018.12.028

## SEEING THE LIGHT (PAGES 64–73)

1. "Cones support alignment to an inconsistent world by suppressing mouse circadian responses to the blue colors associated with twilight." DOI: *https://doi.org/10.1016/j.cub.2019.10.028. 2015.*
2. "Linking light exposure and subsequent sleep: A field polysomnography study in humans." DOI: 10.1093/sleep/zsx165. 2017.
3. "Evening use of light-emitting eReaders negatively affects sleep, circadian timing, and next-morning alertness." a. Departments of Medicine and Neurology, Brigham and Women's Hospital, Boston, MA 02115; b. Division of Sleep Medicine, Harvard Medical School, Boston, MA 02115; and c. Institute of Aerospace Medicine, German Aerospace Center, 51147 Cologne, Germany. Edited by Joseph S. Takahashi, Howard Hughes Medical Institute, University of Texas Southwestern Medical Center, Dallas, TX, and approved November 26, 2014 (received for review September 24, 2014).
4. "Combinations of bright light, scheduled dark, sunglasses, and melatonin to facilitate circadian entrainment to night shift work." *Journal of Biological Rhythms.* 2003 Dec; 18(6):513-23.
5. "Effects of lights of different color temperature on the nocturnal changes in core temperature and melatonin in humans." *Journal of Physiological Anthropology.* 1996, September; 15(5):243-246.
6. "Social jetlag: misalignment of biological and social time." https://pubmed.ncbi.nlm.nih.gov/16687322/

## BEDITATION (PAGES 74–85)

1. This term was most likely coined by Laurence Shorter, author of *The Lazy Guru's Guide to Life*, Orion. 2016.
2. Nelson, J., & Harvey, A. G. (2002). "The differential functions of imagery and verbal thought in insomnia." *Journal of Abnormal Psychology*, 111(4), 665–669. *https://doi.org/10.1037/0021-843X.111.4.665*
3. Broomfield. Niall M. & Espie, Colin A (2003). "Putative Mechanisms Using Subjective and Actigraphic Measurement Of Sleep." *Behavioural and Cognitive Psychotherapy*, 31(3), 313–324. *https://doi.org/10.1017/S1352465803003060*

## TAMING THE MIND (PAGES 86–95)

1. "Duration and timing of sleep are associated with repetitive negative thinking." *Cognitive Therapy and Research* volume 39 *https://link.springer.com/article/10.1007/s10608-014-9651-7*
2. "High intention to fall asleep causes sleep fragmentation." *Journal of Sleep Research*, 2014.
3. American Psychological Association (APA), Stress in America Survey (2013) *https://www.apa.org/news/press/releases/stress/2013/sleep*
4. "Impact of short- and long-term mindfulness meditation training on amygdala reactivity to emotional stimuli." *Neuroimage.* 2018 Nov 1;181:301-313. DOI: 10.1016/j.neuroimage.2018.07.013. Epub 2018 Jul 7.

## GENTLE MOVEMENT (PAGES 96–101)

1. "Exercise and sleep in community-dwelling older adults: evidence for a reciprocal relationship." *Journal of Sleep Research.* 2014 Feb; 23(1):61-8. doi: 10.1111/jsr.12078. Epub 2013 Aug 24. *https://www.ncbi.nlm.nih.gov/pubmed/23980920*
2. National Sleep Foundation.
3. "A before and after comparison of the effects of forest walking on the sleep of a community-based sample of people with sleep complaints." *BioPsychoSocial Medicine.* 2011; 5: 13.
4. *https://rowlandearthing.co.uk/pages/science*

## FEEDING YOUR SLEEP (PAGES 102–117)

1. "Effects of short-term modified fasting on sleep patterns and daytime vigilance in non-obese subjects." (2003 study).
2. Department of Psychology, University of Wisconsin, Madison 53706. 1994. "The relation between cigarette smoking and sleep disturbance." Wetter DW1, Young TB.
3. "Effects of L-Theanine Administration on Stress-Related Symptoms and Cognitive Functions in Healthy Adults: A Randomized Controlled Trial." 2019. *https://www.ncbi.nlm.nih.gov/pmc/articles/PMC6836118/*
4. "The mediating role of sleep in the fish consumption—cognitive functioning relationship: a cohort study." *https://www.ncbi.nlm.nih.gov/pmc/articles/PMC5740156/*

## COMPLEMENTARY AND ALTERNATIVE THERAPIES (PAGES 118–147)

1. "Efficacy and Safety of Ashwagandha (*Withania somnifera*) Root Extract in Insomnia and Anxiety: A Double-blind, Randomized, Placebo-controlled Study." *https://pubmed.ncbi.nlm.nih.gov/31728244/*
2. "Gut modulatory, blood pressure lowering, diuretic, and sedative activities of cardamom." Gilani et al. *https://pubmed.ncbi.nlm.nih.gov/18037596/ https://www.researchgate.net/publication/269560739_Pharmacological_basis_for_the_medicinal_use_of_cardamom_in_asthma*
3. "Drug-use pattern of Chinese herbal medicines in insomnia: a 4-year survey in Taiwan Province of China." *https://doi.org/10.1111/j.1365-2710.2009.01038.x*
4. "Clinical study on acupuncture for primary insomnia." *Journal of Acupuncture and Tuina Science.* 15. 410-414. 10.1007/s11726-017-1037-4. *https://www.researchgate.net/publication/321943491_Clinical_study_on_acupuncture_for_primary_insomnia*
5. "Single Cupping Therapy Session Improves Pain, Sleep, and Disability in Patients with Nonspecific Chronic Low Back Pain." *https://doi.org/10.1016/j.jams.2019.11.004 https://www.sciencedirect.com/science/article/pii/S2005290119302006#sec3*

6. "Effect of Gua Sha Therapy on Perimenopausal Syndrome: A Randomized Controlled Trial." *https://pubmed.ncbi.nlm.nih.gov/27760084/*
7. "Effectiveness of Acupressure for Residents of Long-Term Care Facilities with Insomnia." *https://www.ncbi.nlm.nih.gov/pubmed/20056221*
8. "Scientific Evidence-Based Effects of Hydrotherapy on Various Systems of the Body." *https://www.ncbi.nlm.nih.gov/pmc/articles/PMC4049052/#ref30*
9. "Benefits of Thalassotherapy with Sleep Management on Mood States and Well-being, and Cognitive and Physical Capacities in Healthy Workers." Mounir Chennaoui, et al. Institut de Recherche Biomédicale des Armées (IRBA), Université Paris Descartes—December 3, 2018; Published December 10, 2018
10. "Skin Hunger Helps Explain Your Desperate Longing for Human Touch." *Wired* magazine. *https://www.wired.co.uk/article/skin-hunger-coronavirus-human-touch*

## SOUND ASLEEP (PAGES 148–159)

1. "Acoustic Enhancement of Sleep Slow Oscillations and Concomitant Memory Improvement in Older Adults." 2017. Papalambros NA1, Santostasi G1, Malkani RG1, Braun R2, Weintraub S3, Paller KA4, Zee PC1.
2. "Brain Responses to a 6-Hz Binaural Beat: Effects on General Theta Rhythm and Frontal Midline Theta Activity." 2017, Jun 28. Nantawachara Jirakittayakorn and Yodchanan Wongsawat
3. "The music that helps people sleep and the reasons they believe it works: A mixed methods analysis of online survey reports." Tabitha Trahan, Simon J. Durrant, Daniel Müllensiefen, Victoria J. Williamson, November 14, 2018.
4. *https://www.mattressadvisor.com/sounds-to-fall-asleep/*
5. The findings, presented at the Sleep and Breathing Conference 2015—Silas Daniel Raj— European Respiratory Society (ERS). Abstract Title: "Risk of obstructive sleep apnea in wind musicians." Presentation Date: Tuesday, June 9. Category: Sleep Disorders—Breathing. Abstract ID: 0715.

## HEALING PLANTS (PAGES 160–169)

1. Double-blind study of a valerian preparation, *Pharmacology Biochemistry and Behavior.* 1989 Apr; 2(4):1065-6. *https://www.ncbi.nlm.nih.gov/pubmed/2678162*

## SLEEP TECH (PAGES 176–187)

1. "Electrical stimulation of reward sites in the ventral tegmental area increases dopamine transmission in the nucleus accumbens of the rat." Department of Psychology, University of British Columbia, Canada. 1993.
2. *https://www.sleepfoundation.org/articles/these-mouth-exercises-may-help-stop-snoring*

# ACKNOWLEDGMENTS

There are many people I would like to thank—all those who gave me support on my personal journey to sleep and those directly or indirectly helping me become a sleep ambassador. Thank you . . .

- Mitchell and Jeannette (Mom) for your precious help and contribution.

- Ben Mckie for your amazing guidance and advice.

- Dr. Neil Stanley for your incredible academic knowledge and advocacy.

- Dr. Baoxia Li for practicing Chinese medicine as wisdom and medical art.

- Peter Cox for sharing the power of nutritional healing.

- Dr. Helen Johnson for your down-to-earth healing and coaching.

- Kata and Venetia Armitage for your support and inspiration in the healing of the body and the mind.

- Dr. Aparna Padmanabhan, Dr. Abhishek Joshi, and Kyona Beatty for enlightening me with your expert knowledge of Ayurveda.

- S. N. Goenka for your life-changing teachings and wisdom.

- Gerardo R., Georgia G., Lisa S., Vanessa P., Sophie M., Stacey L., Tessa M., and Daryl F. from my Escape The City tribe for understanding and supporting my vision.

- Chris Pinner for your help, collaboration, and inspiration.

- The Quarto Group team—Eszter, Anna, Kate, Dawn, Martina, Rachel, and Esther—for a superb collaboration.

- Tia, Damola, Siobhan, Shirlene, Risa, and Graham for your help, support, and collaboration.

- Eve Buigues for making me aware of how much sounds impact sleep and for the wonderful soundtracks to my sleep sessions.

*More info at www.thenaturalsleeper.com*